Believe Train Nourish Achieve

A holistic guide to health and wellbeing

Mandy Chandler, Jo Black, Johnny Black

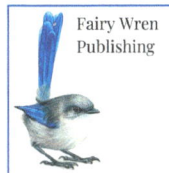

Fairy Wren
Publishing

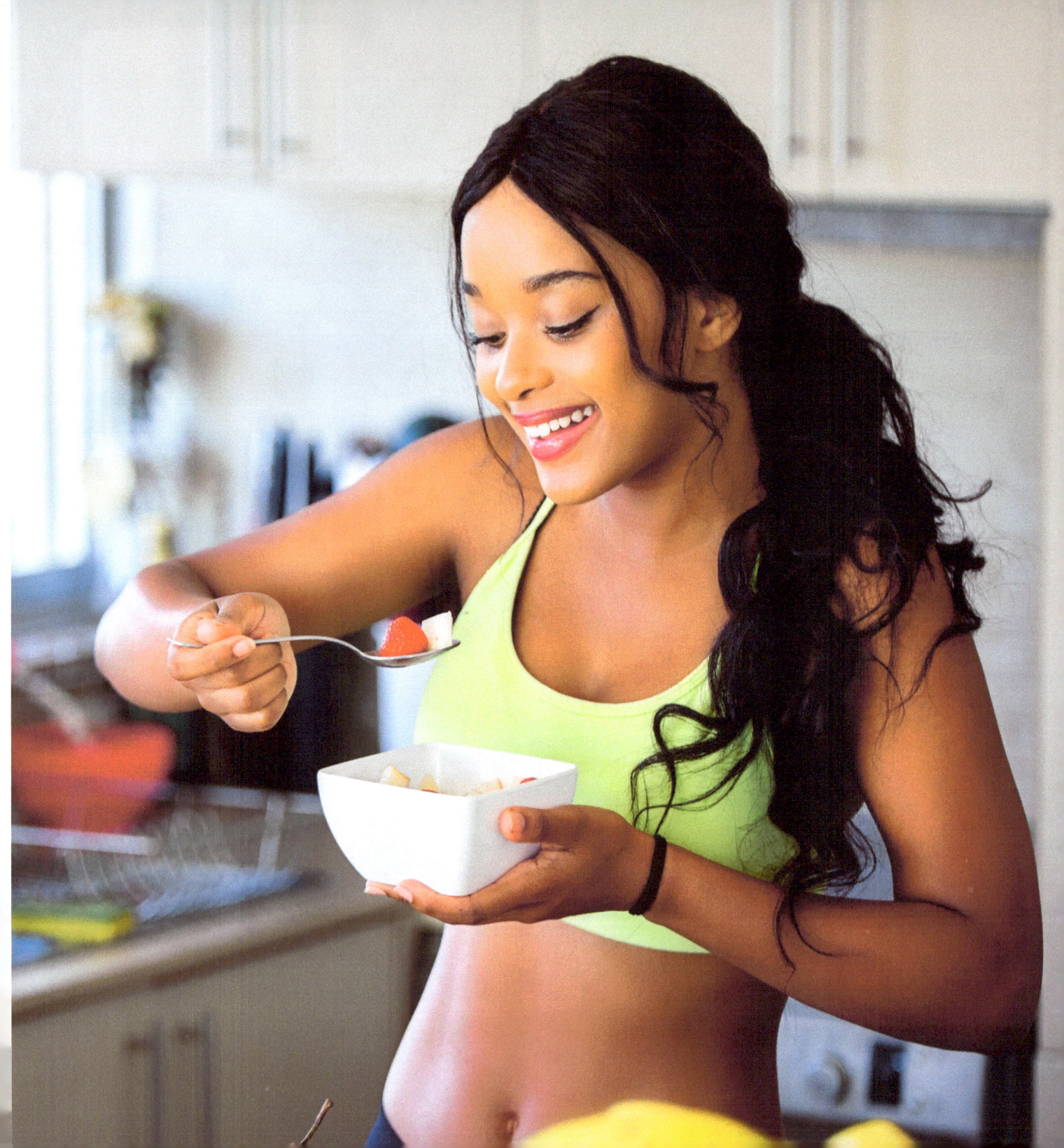

Believe
Train
Nourish
Achieve

A holistic guide to health and wellbeing

First Edition

Published in Brisbane Australia in 2022 by Fairy Wren Publishing

ISBN (Print): 978-0-6455934-0-2   ISBN (EPUB): 978-0-6455934-1-9

Contact: Jo Black Personal Trainer, Life Coach and Clinical Hypnotherapist

Tel. +61 405 907 385 Email: Jo@platinummindandbody.com

NATIONAL LIBRARY OF AUSTRALIA

A catalogue record for this book is available from the National Library of Australia

Disclaimer

The information contained in this book is for educational and informational purposes only and is not intended as medical, mental health or religious advice. Readers must consult a healthcare professional to obtain medical advice relevant to their particular circumstances prior to relying on or otherwise making use of any of the information provided in this book. While we have made every effort to ensure that the information in this book is accurate and informative, we are not medical professionals and the information, including but not limited to text, graphics, images, and other materials, contained in this book, does not take the place of professional or medical advice, diagnosis or treatment. We do not provide any guarantees and assume no legal liability or responsibility for the accuracy, currency or completeness of the information. The authors are not liable for any risks, injury, loss, damage or issues associated with using/acting upon the information herein.

TABLE OF CONTENTS

WELCOME

If you've been searching for practical tools that will help you to overcome fear, gain confidence and become the best possible version of yourself, this book is for you.

Drawing on our holistic approach to health and wellbeing, we have created a practical guide that spans the spectrum of topics from mindfulness and goal setting, training, and nutrition, through to reviewing your progress and rewarding yourself for what you've achieved.

Within these pages, you will find an inspiring collection of useful advice and easy-to-follow practices that will help you to live your best life.

All proceeds from book sales will be donated to Rosie's Friends on the Street. So, thank you for purchasing this book and supporting a cause that is close to our hearts.

We hope you enjoy the book and, if you have any questions or would like to know more, please don't hesitate to reach out to us.

Mandy, Jo & Johnny

www.platinummindandbody.com

MEET THE AUTHORS

Mandy Chandler

Mandy Chandler is a professional writer and editor with over 20 years of experience and a passion for writing about personal development, health, beauty, food, and fitness.

A lifelong student, Mandy's qualifications include an MSc in Chemistry and a Postgraduate Certificate in Editing and Publishing.

When she's not writing or editing, Mandy is a dedicated runner and has completed two ultramarathons, seven marathons, and loads of half-marathons. She has also completed several triathlons, including an Olympic distance triathlon.

To find out more about Mandy's writing and editing services, visit www.mandychandler.com (writing) and www.thebluepencilediting.com (editing) or email: hello@mandychandler.com.

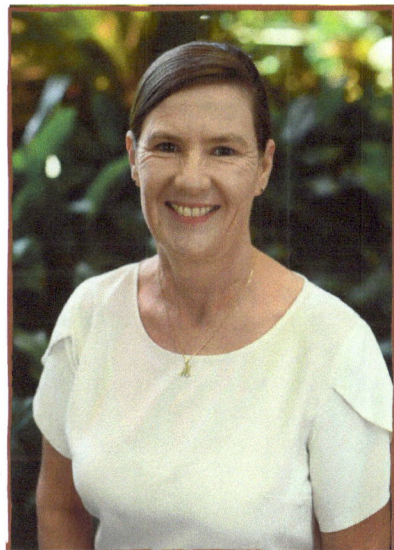

Jo and Johnny Black

Jo and Johnny are founders and owners of the Platinum Mind and Body wellness centre. As fitness professionals, they are passionate about helping people to achieve their goals and optimise all aspects of their physical, emotional and mental health and wellbeing.

To find out how Jo and Johnny can help you live your best life, visit www.platinummindandbody.com.

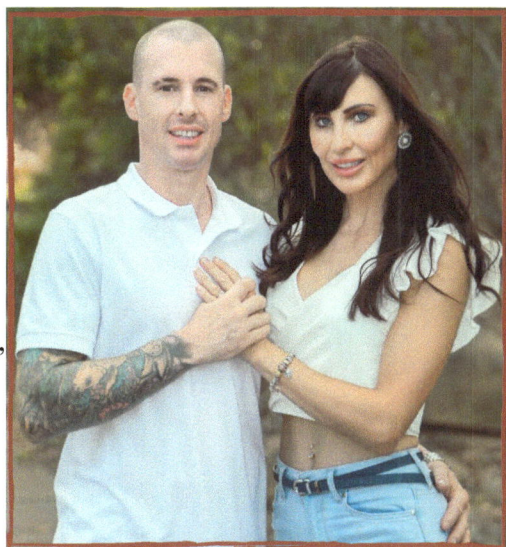

MEET THE FITNESS PROFESSIONALS

Jo Black

Jo is a highly qualified and experienced personal trainer, certified Life Coach (ICF Approved), and Neuro-Linguistic Programming Practitioner. She holds a Diploma of Clinical Hypnosis and Strategic Psychotherapy from the Institute of Applied Psychology and is certified in Timeline Therapy ®.

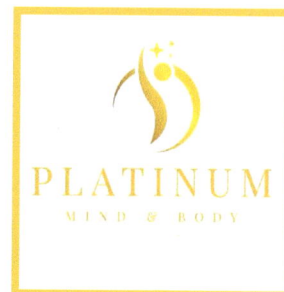

Jo is a member of the International Institute for Complementary Therapists and the Australian Association of Clinical Hypnotherapy and Psychotherapy Inc. as well as the Hypnotherapy Council of Australia. For more information, please visit www.platinummindandbody.com or email jo@platinummindandbody.com.

Johnny Black

Johnny is a qualified nutritionist and health and wellness coach. Over the past 25 years, Johnny has applied his extensive knowledge of sports and nutrition in boxing and fitness gyms, helping his clients to achieve success in boxing and boxing fitness. He provides high-performance training for elite athletes, including Australian national championship winners and Commonwealth Games contenders. For more information, please visit www.warriorboxinggym.com or email Johnny@warriorboxinggym.com.

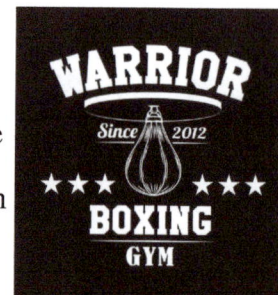

Believe

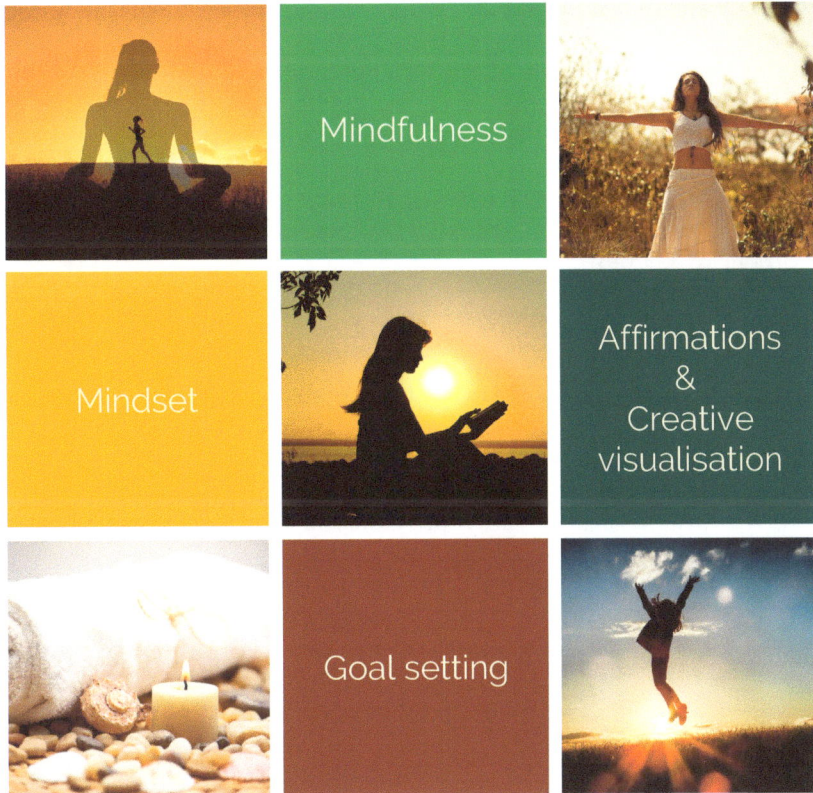

Mindfulness

Mindset

Affirmations & Creative visualisation

Goal setting

"When mind, body, and spirit are in harmony, happiness is the natural result.

Deepak Chopra

If you've come to this book feeling overwhelmed by all the demands of life, frustrated that as hard as you try, you never seem to quite get around to doing the things you love, let alone achieving your dreams; if you're stressed out, anxious, exhausted, and at the end of your tether, this book is especially for you.

We're going to share some practical strategies that will help you to reconnect with your inner self, balance your mind and body, and finally experience that elusive inner peace everyone seems to be banging on about, but no one seems to know where to find.

We've entitled this section, Believe, because it's a simple fact that to succeed in any goal in life: first, you must believe it, then you must be it, and only then will you achieve it.

In this section, we'll provide you with strategies to build the focus, resilience and confidence you need to thrive. We'll share ways in which you can develop the habit of soaking up the joy in each day (mindfulness) and cultivate powerful positive attitudes and thought patterns (mindset) that will naturally lead to success.

As you work through the sections on affirmations, creative visualisation, self-hypnosis, and goal setting, you'll be surprised how easy they are to implement. Don't be fooled by their simplicity though, these are highly effective devices that will help you build a life that you will love.

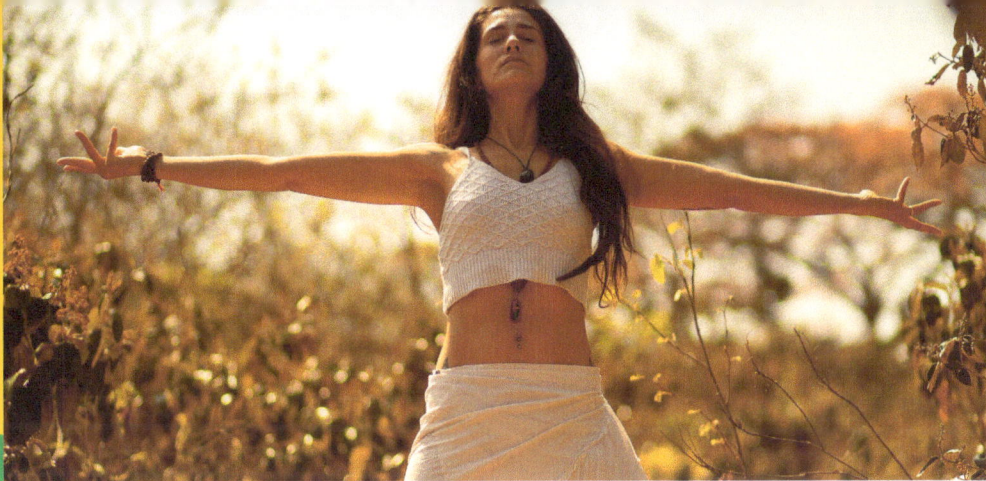

Mindfulness

Life is what happens to us while we are making other plans.
Allen Saunders

Life is fragile. It can change in an instant, and sometimes, those changes can be so dramatic that our lives become almost unrecognisable – even to ourselves. This inherent fragility of life makes it all the more important for us to cherish each and every moment.

All too often, instead of appreciating the moment, we're doing one thing while planning or thinking about the next. We take the kids to the park, but instead of being present and enjoying our time with them, we're on our phones checking emails, scrolling through social media posts, arranging catchups with friends, or planning what we're going to make for dinner. Our fast-paced lives can easily overwhelm us to such an extent that all the joy of living is sapped right out of us.

When we live mindfully, our focus shifts away from future plans and past regrets toward full appreciation and immersion in each and every moment. By living fully in the moment, you'll be able to reduce anxiety and overwhelm and find fulfilment in your life.

Mindfulness is not about being foolishly optimistic, but it is about seeking out the moments of joy in each day and drawing on these moments to see you through the bad times and make the good times even better.

How to be present and find joy in each moment

If you're feeling overwhelmed, frustrated, and depressed, wondering how you could possibly summon up the energy to be fully present. Don't worry. The secret to drawing more energy into your life and being more mindful is simple – pause and look for the joy in every moment.

It doesn't take much energy to pause when something has made you smile and just relish the moment. And, by doing so you will feel more energised and, well, joyful. Plus, later on when your energy flags, you can recall that moment and the joy you felt, and you'll feel energised all over again.

How to live more mindfully

1. Set your intentions for the day – each and every day

What is it that you plan to do today? What would you like to be able to say about who you are and how would you like to feel about how you live your life? Jot the answers down in your journal while you sip your morning coffee. Focus on things that are positive and achievable in one day.

2. Be actively on the lookout for things that give you joy every day

Tune in and take note of the simple joys such as finding a parking space, meeting a friend for coffee, or watching a beautiful sunset. When one of these joyful moments comes along, make a point of absorbing the moment and committing it to memory. In some cases, you might be tempted to take a snapshot with your phone to preserve the moment. That's fine, as long as you take a mental snapshot first. By relying solely on your phone, you'll likely miss out on the depth of the experience you'll get by taking time to mentally pause and relish the moment. Be sure to attach as much emotion and sensory detail (aromas, sensations, sounds, tastes, colours) to the mental snapshot as possible.

3. Take five (or ten) minutes for yourself each day

Read a book or flip through a magazine while you sip a cup of tea or coffee. Go for a ten-minute walk early in the morning before everyone else wakes up. Take a dip in the pool. Close your eyes and relax in a spa or bubble bath. You get the idea.

4. Forget about multitasking – focus on one thing at a time

Multitasking only works when you're using your mind for one task while your hands are engaged in doing something menial that requires little or no brainpower. For example, listening to a podcast while walking the dog. Trying to do two or more tasks that require brainpower, such as answering emails during an important meeting, simply does not work. Instead of being split evenly over the two tasks, your mind repeatedly flips from one task to the other, resulting in neither task being done particularly well. Plus, your poor brain will feel wrung out by the end of it all.

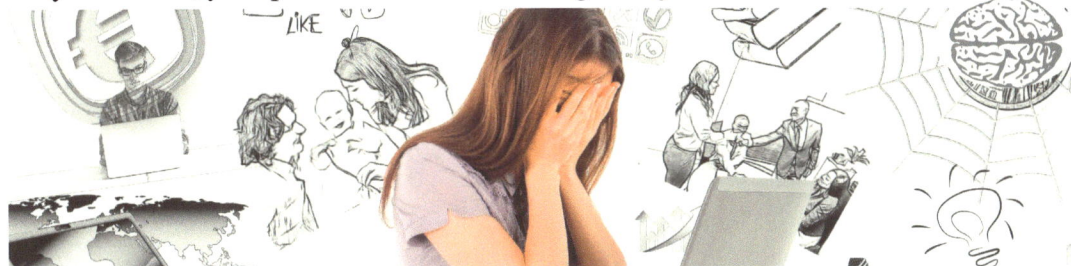

5. Give 100% to what you're doing at the time

Whether you're at work, parenting, partnering or being a friend, give 100% of your attention to the task you're required to perform when you're doing it. If it's in your life and important to you, it's worthy of your full attention.

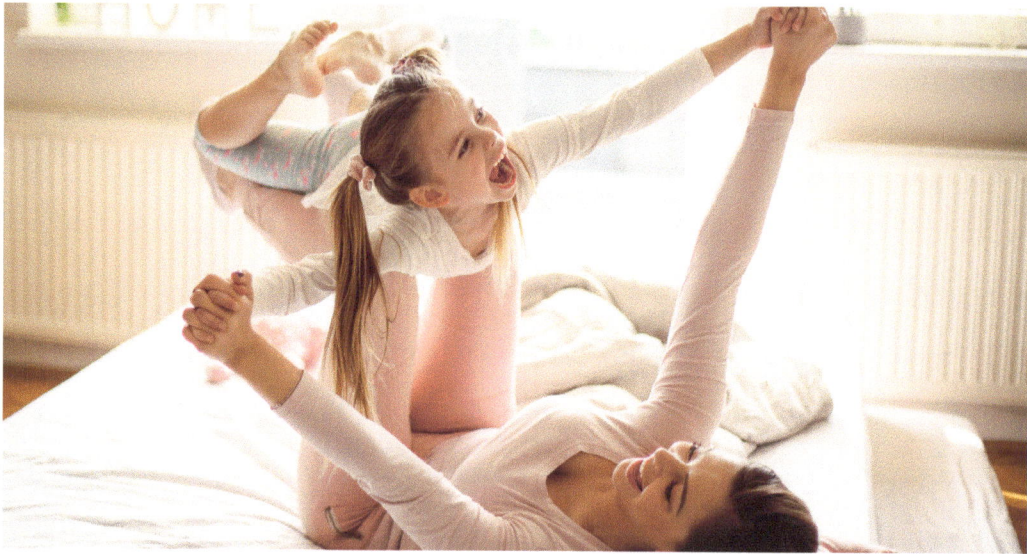

6. Make time to give quality attention to your circle

Don't wait for the right time. Instead, block out time in your schedule to spend with friends and family. This quality time should be sacred, and during these times, your full attention should be focused on the person you're with. For example, rather than checking your emails while on a date night, put your phone aside and give your partner your full attention. This simple act could make a world of difference to your relationship.

At work, your focus should be on your clients and the tasks you need to perform. Keeping one eye on your social media feed while you try to work will affect the quality of your work. Plus, it deprives those you are working with – whether they're bosses, colleagues, clients or students – of your best attention.

Whenever you're interacting with people, make sure your body language aligns with your intention to fully engage. Stand still, turn away from distractions and towards the person. Make eye contact and focus on the person while interacting with them.

7. Be honest about what you need to focus on

Don't be afraid to be honest and tell people when you're unable to give them the attention they deserve. For example, if a friend calls for a chat when you're under pressure at work, don't try to divide your attention between the phone call and your work. Instead, politely explain that you have a deadline and suggest a catch-up at a more convenient time. This will leave your friend feeling acknowledged and respected rather than being rushed or brushed off. And you'll be able to meet that deadline.

> **"** You should sit in meditation for twenty minutes every day unless you're too busy – on those days you should sit for an hour.
>
> Dr. Sukhraj Dhillon

8. Spend time in silence every day

Whether it's five minutes or twenty, the value of spending time in silence each day cannot be underestimated. It's up to you whether you spend these minutes meditating, jogging/walking (without earphones), simply sitting in a comfy chair or even lying down. The important thing is to be still, stay silent, switch off from your surroundings, relax and allow your mind to wander uncensored.

This practice helps you to release tension, unwind, and process your day. If you'd like to spend this time meditating, there are some great apps that can help you to get started, but all you really need to do (at least initially) is to sit comfortably, focus on your breathing, and let your thoughts come and go.

Try not to hold onto any one thought – just acknowledge them and let them float away. If you find yourself latching onto a thought and getting carried away, simply stop and bring your focus back to your breathing once more. If you're new to the practice, start with shorter sessions of one to five minutes. Set a timer, so you know when the session is over. The more you practice, the easier it will become, and you'll be able to extend your meditations to ten or even twenty minutes, or more.

9. Eating mindfully

Instead of wolfing down your meals at your desk at work or in front of the TV at home, try sitting down at a table and savouring each bite. Put your utensils down between bites, chew your food thoroughly before swallowing, and take the time to experience all the wonderful textures and flavours.

Once you've finished, spend another ten to fifteen minutes at the table, enjoying the company of your family, friends or colleagues, or just relishing a moment to yourself before heading off to take on the rest of your day.

Believe. Train. Nourish. Achieve.

10. Ease up and disconnect at night to recharge your batteries

When you're constantly busy and bombarded 24/7 by information, stimulation, and communication, it can be difficult to slow down and take a break from it all. But it's vital to disconnect, especially at night. The constant demands of notifications, social media scrolling, and obsessive inbox checking make it difficult to rest. Eliminate these, and you'll be able to fully recharge and be more present in everyday life. A good way to do this is to create phone-free zones in your home. Spending time away from your phone will reduce your overall stress levels and improve your energy levels, so you can maintain a healthy mind and body.

Quick tip

Mindfulness is about making the most of the life you have right now. You can learn from the past, and you certainly should look toward the future, but true joy comes from focusing on the present and enjoying each moment.

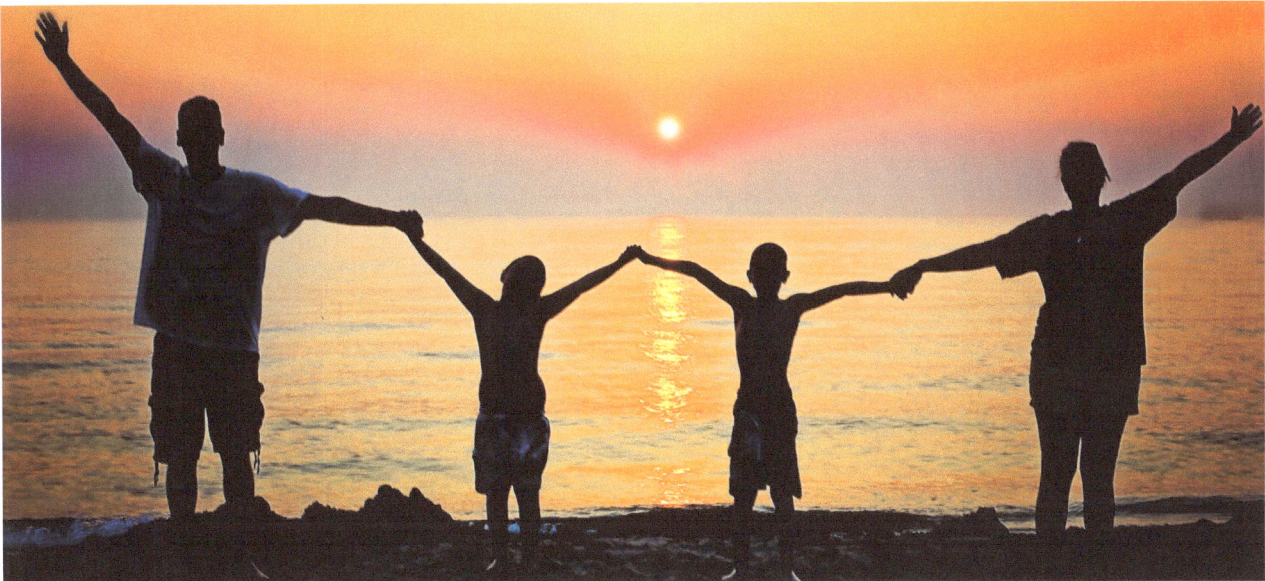

NOTES

Believe. Train. Nourish. Achieve.

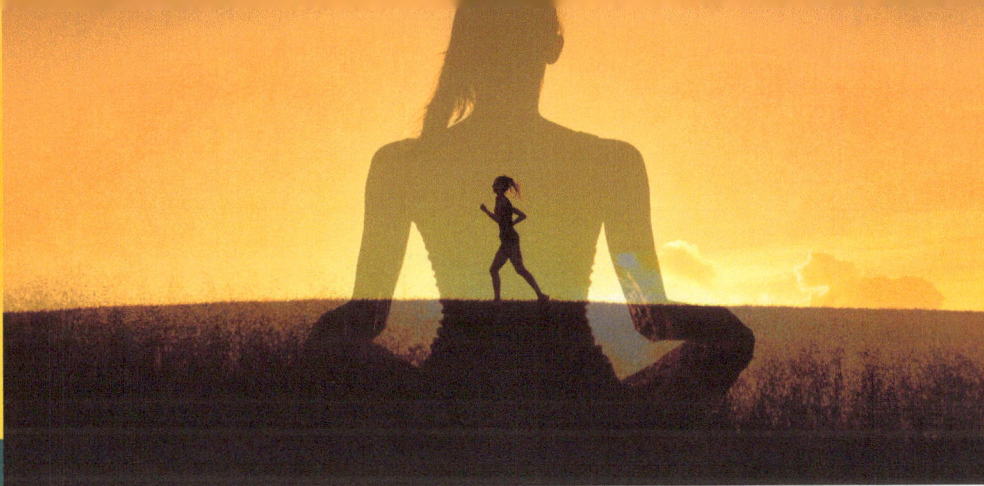

Mindset

Whether you think you can or you think you can't. You're right.

Henry Ford

Your journey to health and wellbeing will include plenty of fun times, happy moments, achievements, celebrations, fulfillment, and rewards. But it won't all be plain sailing. There'll be times when you'll be required to dig deep in order to achieve your dreams. A good mindset will provide the mental and emotional strength you need to push through the tough times and achieve your goals.

All change begins in the mind

There are six crucial mindset shifts you'll need to make to build a winning mentality and start living your best life.

Mindset shift #1 You can start whenever you want

There's no reason to wait for the calendar to tell you when it's okay to start. You don't need to wait for next week, next month or next year. You can start today – even if it is Thursday!

Mindset shift #2 You don't need to make resolutions ever again

Forget resolutions. They're so last year. Resolutions are all about the things that you think you should change in your life. They are motivated by external factors, such as social pressures and norms. It's time to kick them to the curb and create a set of intentions instead.

Intentions are about "can" and "will", rather than "should". They're deeply personal because they are based on your values (the things that are important to you) and not on the demands that society places on you. They are about who you want to be and how you want to be living at the end of this month, this quarter, this year or this period of your choosing.

When you've set your intentions, you'll be able to stop struggling with the things you think you should be doing and start doing the things that are really important to you.

Here's a quick example:

A resolution might be: *I want to lose weight so people don't stare at me when I go to the beach this summer.*

An intention would be: *It's important to me to be fit and healthy so I can be there for my kids. So, I'm committed to eating healthy foods and exercising for half an hour each day.*

Mindset shift #3 Explore what really matters to you

The first step in setting your intentions is to discover the things that are truly important to you. It's easy to get caught up in the "busyness" of life, never able to find the time for the things that really matter, such as spending time with loved ones, working on your health and fitness, or pursuing creative endeavours.

In this mindset shift, we're asking you to change your focus from everyday "busyness" to make time for the things that really matter to you. But how do you know what really matters? Surely jobs, shopping, social engagements, and everything else that goes with modern life are important? They may be, but we want you to take a moment and dig a little deeper to find out what's *really* important to you.

The things that matter most to you will resonate with your values

Not sure about what your values are? You're not alone. Most people never really take the time to put their values into words. It's not hard to do, though.

Simply take some time to ask yourself, 'What is really important to me?' Then jot down your answers without censoring them. There are no right or wrong answers.

And remember, none of these things reflect on your value as a person. It really doesn't matter at all whether you value top achievement in your career, living a luxurious lifestyle, driving a fancy car, or whether you place no value at all on material possessions. Just be as unapologetically honest as possible and write down everything that comes to mind.

Once you've got it all down, try to prioritise your list, so you have your most important values at the top and the rest listed in descending order of importance to you. Again, remember there is no right or wrong here.

At this point, you probably have a list that includes some (or all) of the following: my family, my health, my career, my car, my house, my reputation, and so on. That's great. The top five or six values on your list will represent your core values – the things that matter most to you.

Next, you need to get really specific about the things that make up each of your core values. For example, if your health is important to you, what aspects of it are most important to you? Is it to be stronger and fitter? To be able to run a half marathon? To be fit enough to keep up with your kids? Or is it to have more energy so you can cope with your demanding career?

Write a value statement for each of your core values that describes in detail exactly what it is about each value is important to you. These value statements should be deeply personal reflections of what each value means to you.

WHAT IS REALLY IMPORTANT TO ME?

Believe. Train. Nourish. Achieve.

MY VALUE STATEMENTS

Making decisions can be exhausting. In fact, scientists have proven that after a full day of decision-making, your brain becomes fatigued and unable to cope with further decisions. There's even a name for this – it's called *decision fatigue*.

Avoiding decision fatigue is a strategy used by many successful people, including Bill Gates, Richard Branson, Mark Zuckerberg, Steve Jobs, and Barack Obama. These high achievers are notorious for wearing the same thing every day – their reasoning being that it's one less daily decision they need to make, and they can save that energy to make the really important decisions their careers require.

Now, we're not suggesting you change your wardrobe. But, once you know what's important to you, you will waste a lot less energy making decisions.

Here's why:

When you know your values, you approach decisions from a different point of view. Instead of asking 'Which option is better?' you'll be asking 'Which option fits best with my values and what I'm trying to achieve?'

So, instead of wasting energy making endless lists of pros and cons for each option, you'll be able to simply examine how well each option suits your needs and make your decision on that basis.

For example, imagine a simple scenario where you have to choose between an apple or an orange. Using our method of value-based decision-making, you won't be comparing apples and oranges to discover which is the better fruit. Instead, you'll be asking 'Which fruit best suits my current requirements?' So, if what you need is a thirst quenching fruit, the question becomes which fruit is the juiciest, in which case the orange is the clear winner. Problem solved!

Here's another example. Imagine you want to get a distinction in your studies, and you've been invited a party on the night before the exam.

Weighing up a night out against a night of studying is hardly going to lead you to the best choice. But, a value-based decision-making process makes things a lot easier. Instead of asking 'Which would I rather do?' you'll be asking 'Does going to the party get me closer to (or further from) what I value, which in this case, is getting a distinction in my exam?' Suddenly, the right option is crystal clear, and choosing to stay home and study becomes easier. This type of thinking allows you to reframe the situation in a way that empowers you: you're not staying home because you *have to*, you're doing it because *you* want to get that distinction.

Reviewing your options against your values, rather than against each other, may even reveal new alternatives, such as a watermelon, instead of an apple or an orange, if you're after a juicy fruit.

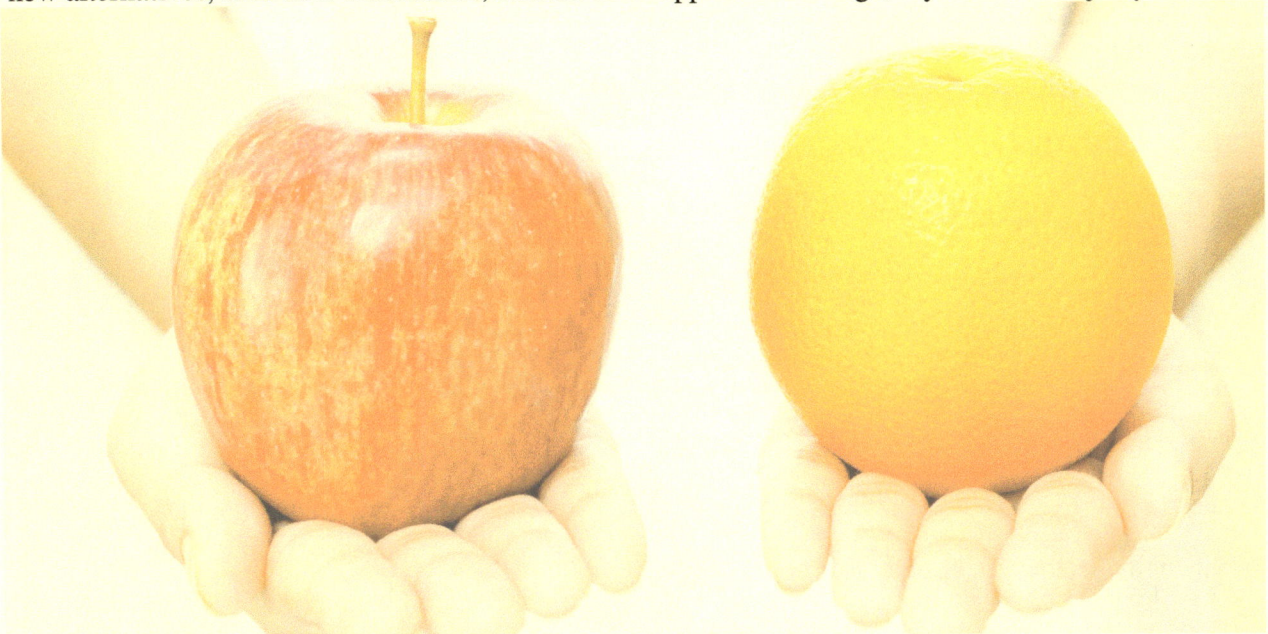

Mindset shift #4 Be brave enough to ask how your current lifestyle measures up against your values

Now that you're clear on your core values, it's time to be brave and take stock of your current lifestyle. How does your life right now align with your values? Don't be disheartened if you discover that there's a wide gap between your life and your values. The work you're doing here might be confronting, but it is also life-changing. And, noticing the gap between your current lifestyle and your values might provide the motivation you need to take action.

A potential pitfall here is that you might feel pressurised to make a million changes all at once. Don't. Trying to change everything all at once will only leave you feeling frustrated, overwhelmed, disappointed, and wrung out.

It takes time and commitment to make changes in your life, and they're best approached slowly and carefully. Focus on making small but significant changes over time. These changes will be easier to achieve and will help to motivate you to keep going.

Incremental improvement is the key to success. And, as Maya Angelo said, 'Success breeds success.' So, by achieving these small changes, you'll be encouraged to make even more changes until, eventually, you begin to see your values reflected in the life you have created.

Mindset shift #5 Review, refresh and recommit to your values every six months

Reviewing your life against your core values will allow you to identify any changes you need to make and highlight those areas where you may have gone off track. Don't forget to celebrate your successes and try to find the lessons in your mistakes. We'll go into more detail about how to do all of this in the Achieve section of this book.

Gratitude

Gratitude has become a buzzword of the modern age with everyone from the Dalai Lama to TV talk show hosts extolling the benefits of the gratitude mindset. But, far from being just another abstract self-help fad, gratitude practices have been scientifically validated as effective tools that can significantly improve your quality of life.

Research findings published in leading psychology and psychiatry journals point to significant mental and physical benefits, including a strong positive correlation between gratitude, happiness, and emotional resilience. Studies have shown that suicidal patients and people battling terminal diseases felt more hopeful and positive after writing gratitude letters.

Gratitude practices have helped people to overcome depression, insomnia, substance abuse, eating disorders, anxiety, and burnout. It has also been linked to significant reductions in cardiac disease, inflammation, and neurodegeneration.

What this means is that, when you take time to stop and appreciate the things that are valuable and meaningful to you and express your thankfulness for having these things in your life, you're cultivating a powerful mindset of gratitude that, with regular practice, over time, delivers a multitude of benefits, including reduced stress, enhanced mood, improved sleep-wake cycles, greater health, stronger immune response, and better interpersonal relationships.

So, what's the best way to cultivate an attitude of gratitude?

Thanks to neuroplasticity, it's easy for us to train our brains to develop and maintain an attitude of gratitude. What's neuroplasticity? Well, it's really just a fancy term that describes your brain's ability to rewire itself whenever you learn a new skill.

Take riding a bicycle for example. The saying goes that you never forget how to ride a bicycle. Once you've learnt the skill required, you can simply hop on and pedal away – even if it's been years or decades since you last rode.

This is because when you learnt to ride, your brain rewired itself to include pathways that allow you to link the thoughts and actions required to ride your bike. With practice, these new pathways became more firmly established, making it easier and easier to ride your bike, until eventually, you could do it without thinking.

It's the same with gratitude. The more you practice gratitude, the more your brain becomes wired toward it. It becomes easier to feel grateful, and over time, gratitude becomes your brain's default setting. This means you get to experience all those wonderful benefits that gratitude brings to your life every day – without very much effort at all.

Gratitude is NOT the same as wishful thinking

Contrary to what "pop" psychology preaches about manifesting your desires and eliminating unpleasant things from your life; gratitude is not a magic wand that can be waved around at will to make life plain sailing.

Life will always have ups and downs and throw curve balls at you just when you think everything is going fine. Gratitude practices won't stop this, but they will help you to cope better with whatever life throws at you.

Gratitude is also not a miracle overnight cure. It takes commitment, time, and practice to rewire your brain into an attitude of gratitude and maintain that wiring so that it stands up to any upheavals in your life. But it is well worth it.

Gratitude is like a superpower

Instead of removing the bad stuff in your life, gratitude works like a super-power, giving you the ability to overcome obstacles. It enhances the way you experience life – even when bad things happen.

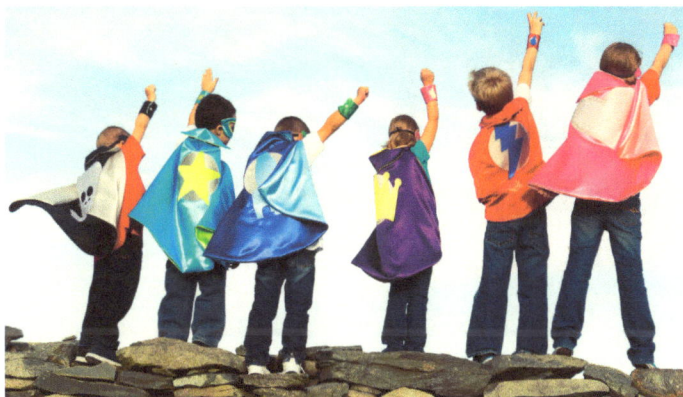

Just like all superheroes, you need to practice using your gratitude superpower until it becomes part of who you are. Once gratitude becomes your default state of mind, you can use it to drive out fear, criticism, depression, self-doubt, and pessimism regardless of your circumstances.

What's more, with a permanent attitude of gratitude, you'll experience life with a greater sense of meaning and purpose, you'll feel more alive, and be more open to the joy and beauty in the world around you. This doesn't mean you see everything through rose-tinted glasses. Instead, you choose to see the good in everything. So that, when isolation, separation, death, illness, and loneliness close in, you're able to keep going and support others.

How to train your mind towards gratitude

Here's a simple gratitude practice that's easy to do and very effective.

Daily gratitude practice

Each morning, while enjoying your favourite morning drink – whether it's tea, coffee or a green smoothie – find a quiet spot, away from the distractions of phones, computers or TVs, and take some time to answer the following questions:

1. What am I grateful for from yesterday?

2. What am I grateful for today?

3. What am I grateful for about tomorrow?

THINGS I AM GRATEFUL FOR

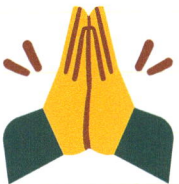

THINGS I AM GRATEFUL FOR

Believe. Train. Nourish. Achieve.

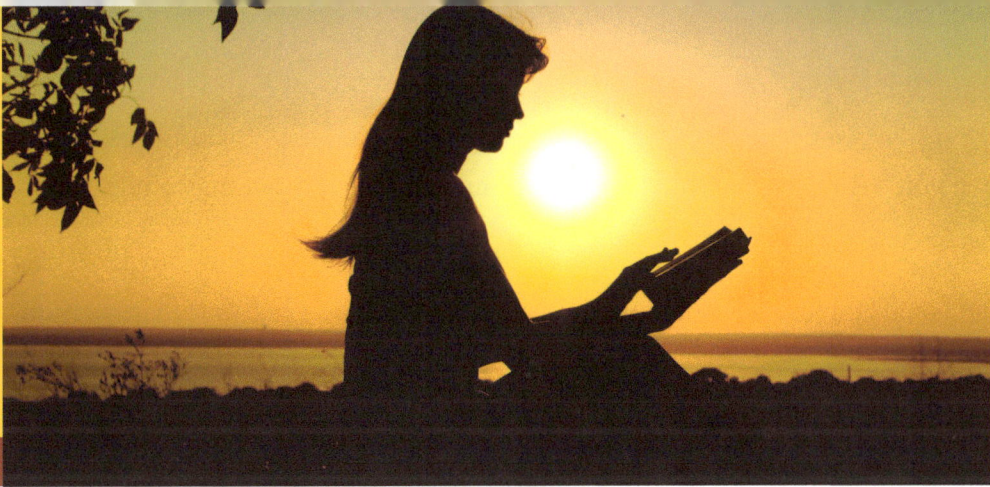

Affirmations

Your words are very powerful, and what you say matters.
Keep them positive and powerful!
Farshad Asl

This chapter comes with one free eye-roll, redeemable by those of you who think affirmations are just a bit too "woo-woo" to work. Go on, get it over with, you know you want to. 😊

Okay, now that's out of the way, let's take a closer look at affirmations, what they are, and why they really do work. No, really.

We've already established that a strong positive and resilient mindset is the key to leading a happy and fulfilling life. Affirmations are the foundation upon which that mindset is built. Let's take a look at how this happens.

It starts with the basic premise that words have power. Don't believe us? Consider this: everything in existence today started out as an idea, a thought, a word.

When you want to create something, anything at all, be it a painting, a bikini body or a better mousetrap, first, you must imagine it, then you put your thoughts and imaginings into words, and only then can you begin to create it in real life.

Affirmations help you to put your deepest desires, thoughts, and imaginings into words. By saying them out loud, you cement them into beliefs and build a mindset that empowers you to create the life you want.

It's true, affirmations have been given a bad rap. But it's not the idea behind affirmations that's faulty, it's how they are taught that's the problem. Over the years, people have been teaching affirmations in ways that simply don't work. Let's look at a few common misconceptions.

Affirmations do not involve lying to yourself

The old-fashioned way of teaching and practicing affirmations involves simply saying what you want to be true over and over again. It is largely responsible for so many people giving up on them altogether or never attempting them in the first place. Here's why.

Saying 'I am a millionaire' over and over again when you're clearly not is never going to make you one. Nor is saying 'I have 6% body fat' over and over again going to make that true for you if it's not.

By saying affirmations, you are activating your subconscious mind. And, your subconscious is pretty smart. So, repeating a bunch of outright lies – no matter how often or for however long you continue to do so – will never convince your subconscious that they are true and will never be the optimal strategy for success.

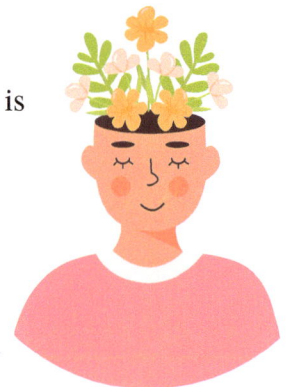

Affirmations do not involve bland statements

Another popular way of teaching affirmations is to have people create and recite bland statements about what they want to happen. For example, 'I am a magnet for money' or 'money constantly flows into my life.'

These affirmations are nothing more than a panacea to make you feel good for a little while, but they cannot improve your financial situation.

In order to be effective, affirmations must articulate your desires clearly, so that your subconscious stands up and takes notice. They should tell it exactly what you want and what you need to do to get it. Such affirmations work because they get your subconscious on board, and it starts motivating you to take the actions that will align your life with your desires. And that's the "magic sauce" that makes affirmations so powerful.

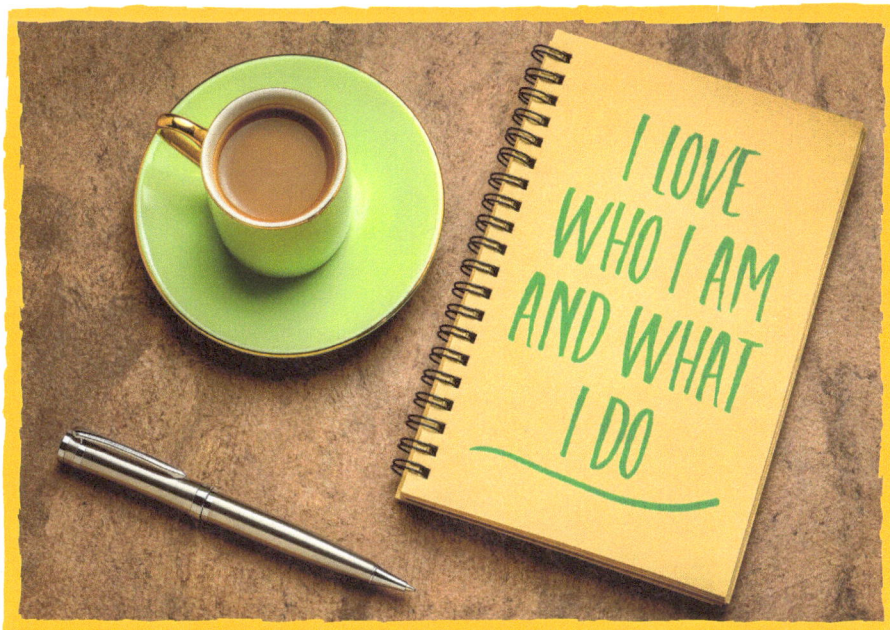

Four steps to creating effective affirmations

Step 1 Create powerful affirmations with as much detail as possible

The formula for an effective affirmation is:

SMART Goal + Self + Action + Why

Start by writing down the extraordinary outcome or SMART goal (a goal that is specific, measurable, achievable, realistic, and time-based – more on this later) you wish to achieve. Don't just write down something you want. Go deeper and think of something you truly desire, and that you are committed to achieving.

For example, if you'd like to get fit, but your true desire is to to run a half marathon, instead of just saying 'I want to get fit' your affirmation would be:

I am 100% committed to running a half marathon in July (SMART goal).

"Self" refers to the person you need to be to achieve this goal. For example, if you're going for a job interview, but you lack self-confidence, you might use the affirmation:

I am 100% committed to succeeding in my job interview today (SMART goal). I believe in, trust, and have confidence in myself, and my ability to answer questions fully and clearly demonstrate my suitability for the role (self).

Wanting something is all fine and well, but nothing will happen without action. Affirmations are no exception. In order for them to work, they need to be accompanied by dedicated and consistent action. So, when formulating your affirmations, you need to include the necessary actions you will take and *when* you will take them – be specific.

For example, if you're starting a new fitness program, you might use the affirmation:

I am 100% committed to completing the 12-week body transformation challenge (SMART goal). I am energized and eager (self) to follow the program, eat well, exercise regularly, and get plenty of rest (actions).

The more specific your affirmations are the better. They should include as much detail about the action you're going to take as possible as well as how much, how often, and for how long you will be taking this action.

For example, if you want to run a half marathon, your affirmation might look something like:

To ensure that I am ready to run my first half marathon in July (SMART goal), I am 100% committed to following my running training program for the next 12 weeks. I trust and believe in myself, and I am confident in my ability (self) to run or cross-train every morning from 5:00 am to 6:00 am, five days a week – no exceptions, no excuses (detailed action).

To strengthen your commitment, don't forget to include your reasons for wanting to achieve this (your why). So, your completed affirmation for the half marathon goal would be:

I am 100% committed to running my first half marathon in July (SMART goal). I believe in, trust, and have confidence in my ability (self) to run or cross-train every morning from 5:00 am to 6:00 am, five days a week – no exceptions, no excuses (action). I am doing this to raise funds for breast cancer research (why).

I am brave I am loved I am kind

Step 2 Say your affirmations out loud every morning

If you're like most of us, you've probably experienced that annoying human phenomenon where you spend the whole weekend making all these great plans for losing weight, getting fitter and healthier or training for that comp you just entered. And, by Monday morning, you've ordered a caramel latte with cream and a choc-chip muffin on your way into the office and made plans to go out with your colleagues after work instead of hitting the gym. It's like all the hours of planning and prepping didn't even happen, and you've entirely forgotten all about the diet, exercise or training plans that you were supposed to put into action today.

This is where saying your affirmations out loud every day can really make all the difference.

It's not magic – just a daily reminder of the path you've chosen and committed to – but it works like magic. That's because the more you remind yourself of your commitment, the more likely you are to follow through with it. By saying your affirmations out loud each day, you're programming your subconscious with the attitudes and mindset you need to get out there and achieve your goals. And, you're ensuring that your conscious mind stays focused on your goals, taking the actions you need to take in order to succeed, and prioritising them over all the distractions and temptations you're going to face during the day.

To get the best results, you must commit to reading your affirmations out loud every day.

Make them part of your routine, just like brushing your teeth. In fact, a great way to work them into your morning routine is to habit-stack them with toothbrushing. This means saying your affirmations as soon as you're done brushing your teeth each day. So, you're less likely to forget.

Step 3 Don't just repeat your affirmations mindlessly

Instead of mouthing your affirmations on autopilot, try to channel the enthusiasm and determination you felt when setting your goals. Aim to experience that excitement all over again as you recite your affirmations. Get your enthusiasm pumping by putting as much authentic emotion into them as you can. Feel the truth of what you're affirming and draw on that positive emotion to stay motivated.

Step 4 Review and revise your affirmations

Your affirmations will grow and change as you progress through life. Each time you have a new intention, goal or dream, you will need to revisit and revise your affirmations to ensure you have the appropriate default mindset with all the necessary components for success.

Quick tip Be on the lookout for inspiring quotes, strategies or ideas that you can add to your affirmations to help build a winning mindset.

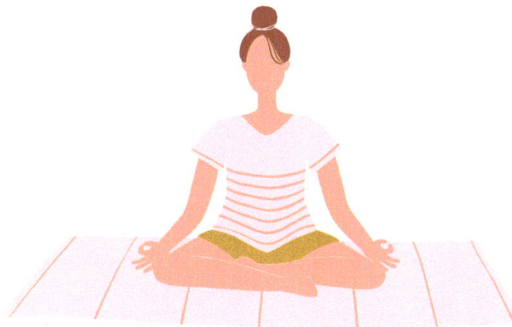

Using affirmations to overcome negative thinking and limiting beliefs

Affirmations program your subconscious mind to believe certain things about yourself and the world around you, and in doing so, they help you to create the reality you want.

You can use affirmations to change your self-talk and replace negative thinking and limiting beliefs with positive beliefs and behaviours. This helps you to be successful in all areas of your life whether in your career, health, fitness, personal relationships or finances. By saying and thinking positive and uplifting things about yourself, you're paving the way to achieving your goals.

By creating affirmations that reflect the sense of self-worth, you're taking a key step on the path to a healthier, happier you. Here are a few ideas you can weave into affirmations to overcome negative thinking, low self-esteem, and limiting beliefs.

- I know, accept, and believe in myself.
- I believe in my dreams and in my ability to achieve them.
- I accept 100% responsibility for my life.
- I am in charge of how I feel, and I choose to be positive today.
- I create happiness and opportunities wherever I go.
- Every day is a fresh start with a new beginning to make my own.
- I am grateful for the life I am creating.
- I am in charge of my happiness.
- Everything I do will lead me to where I need to be.
- I live each day to the fullest.
- I love and accept myself just as I am.

DAILY AFFIRMATIONS & GRATITUDE WORKSHEET

My Affirmations

Today, I look forward to...

How can I set myself up for success?

MORNING

I am grateful for...

I was successful when...

The most wonderful thing that happened today was...

BEDTIME

NOTES

Believe. Train. Nourish. Achieve.

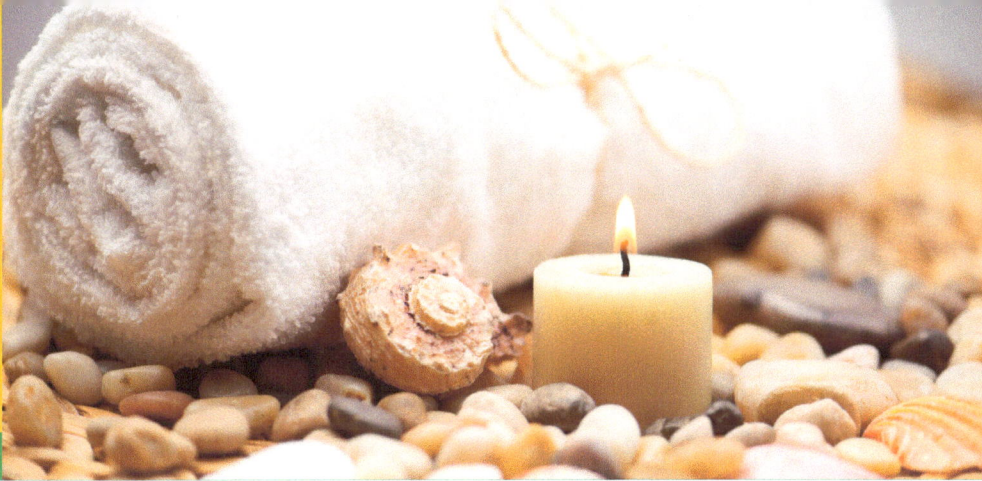

Creative visualisation

Dare to visualize a world in which your
most treasured dreams have come true.

Ralph Marston

Don't judge this chapter by its slightly "new age" title. In it, you'll find out just how powerful and practical visualisations really are – despite the misconceptions surrounding them.

Let's take a look at a common scenario. You've probably experienced something similar at some stage in your life. Imagine you had your eye on a particular car. Maybe your first car or perhaps something fancy like a luxury or sports car. Either way, if you're like most of us, you've probably stared at pictures in magazines, watched the ads on TV, and gazed longingly through showroom windows at your desired make and model. Heck, it may even have replaced your girlfriend as the lock screen image on your mobile (don't worry, we won't tell). Suffice it to say, in those giddy days before it became yours, you probably couldn't stop staring at it.

Then, right around the time when you were getting ready to make the purchase, you suddenly started seeing that exact car – everywhere. Has everyone suddenly purchased *your* dream car? Um, no.

Scientifically speaking, this phenomenon of seeing the object you desire everywhere is an actual thing. It's called *the Baader-Meinhof phenomenon*, and it's a sign that your brain has tuned in to what you've been visualising and dreaming about. Freaky right?

Now, let's backtrack just a little. On any given day, your subconscious mind works in the background filtering out what it thinks is unimportant information and pushing into your conscious mind only those things it thinks are worth noticing.

In fact, it is quite selective when deciding what grabs your attention and what is ignored. Now, there's no need to get grumpy about it. Your subconscious is not censoring you – it's just doing its job, which is to protect you from information overload and help you to concentrate on what's really important – like your dream car, for instance.

So, when you were looking at pictures, making smudge marks on showroom windows, and fantasising about what it would be like to be behind the wheel of that car, you were actually programming your subconscious to take note of it and bring it to your attention whenever it sees one. And that's why you ended up seeing that same car everywhere! The truth is, it's always been there, except your subconscious blocked it out, until by visualising it, you primed your subconscious to give your brain a nudge whenever it saw one.

While visualisation in this example probably happened quite naturally without you deliberately doing it, you can use the same phenomenon to deliberately program your subconscious mind so that it prompts your conscious mind about other things you want to achieve. Called *creative visualisation*, it involves picturing what you want to happen in your mind's eye before it's happened.

With creative visualisation, you're tapping into the brain's natural tendency to focus on the things you visualise. This, in turn, helps you to stay focused on your goal and take the necessary steps to achieve it.

Formulate and stamp indelibly on your mind a mental picture of yourself succeeding. Hold onto this picture tenaciously and never permit it to fade. Your mind will seek to develop this picture.

Dr. Norman Vincent Peale

The science behind creative visualisation

Why does creative visualisation work? Scientific studies indicate that, in addition to leveraging your brain's natural attraction to visual stimuli, there is a certain type of nerve cell in your brain that may play an important role in making visualisation so effective. Known as *mirror neurons*, they allow you to improve your physical abilities not only by watching other people perform tasks but also by visualising yourself doing them. For example, studies have shown that vivid visualisation sessions led to a significant increase in muscle mass in weightlifters, without them actually lifting any weights, and mirror neurons made this possible.

While we don't recommend that you give up on actually doing things and instead try to make things happen just by sitting around visualising, it's well worth adding this highly effective tool to your daily routine.

What should you visualise?

Visualise what your life would be like if you fulfilled your potential

Start by imagining your biggest goals – those things you've always dreamed of doing/ being.

Try to answer these questions:

- What does success look like for you – in terms of lifestyle, career, relationships, and mindset?

- How will it feel?

- Who will you need to be to achieve those goals?

This type of big-picture visualisation is important to keep you focused on the long game, and it will help you keep your eye on the prize when it comes to big overarching goals.

Visualise the daily things that you need to do to get you closer to your goals

If you're only focussing on that one final achievement (e.g., crossing the finish line of your first marathon), you'll have missed out on celebrating all the smaller and equally important victories leading up to it (e.g., your first 5 km, 10 km, half marathon, and so on). That's why it's important to also visualise the daily steps that you need to take to get closer to your bigger goals. By visualising yourself successfully completing these smaller steps each day, you'll be ready and eager to take action and make them happen.

This is especially important early on in the process of pursuing a big goal. For example, when you start training for your first marathon, your daily visualisation should focus on the successful completion of that day's training. Or, if your goal is to lose 15 kg, then your daily visualisation should focus on the healthy meals and snacks you will be eating that day.

Visualise things that are achievable

Whatever you visualise must be within the realm of possibility for you. You should be able to honestly and sensibly observe yourself taking the steps and achieving whatever it is you're visualising. If you're middle-aged and not very fit, for example, you will likely never run a sub-two-hour marathon – no matter how much visualisation you do – simply because this goal is well beyond the reach of most ordinary folk. But, you could visualise yourself completing a 5 km parkrun, and in time, with training, you could achieve this goal.

Visualise what you want to achieve in all areas of your life

Visualisations are not just for fitness goals either, you can use them to prepare for exams, confidently present to clients, succeed at an interview, and achieve all sorts of goals in your personal and professional life, whether it's making partner, writing a novel or learning to play the piano.

Visualise the person you need to be to achieve your goals

The person you have been up to now, with the habits you have, and the choices you make, does not define the person you can become. The person you are now is likely not the person you need to be to achieve your vision. Think about the person you need to become. What type of person will take the necessary steps and turn your dreams into reality? Then visualise becoming that person. How will your choices, habits, and values have to change?

> **Every morning you have two choices: continue to sleep with your dreams or wake up and chase them.** Carmelo Anthony

For example, maybe until now, you've been the type to hit the snooze button several times before getting up and dashing off to work. On the way in, you might habitually swing by your favourite bakery to grab a butterscotch muffin and an iced mocha with cream for breakfast.

Now, if your dream is to complete a 10 km fun run and raise money for breast cancer, you're going to need to make some changes.

You will need to say goodbye (with love and respect) to the snooze-button-pounding, muffin-munching, mocha-latte-slurping version of yourself and visualise a different you. In this case, one that gets out of bed half an hour early to go for a run before it's too hot and then enjoys a healthy breakfast before heading off to work.

Visualisation might feel difficult and uncomfortable at first, but you'll have to get out of your comfort zone if you want to turn your dreams into reality.

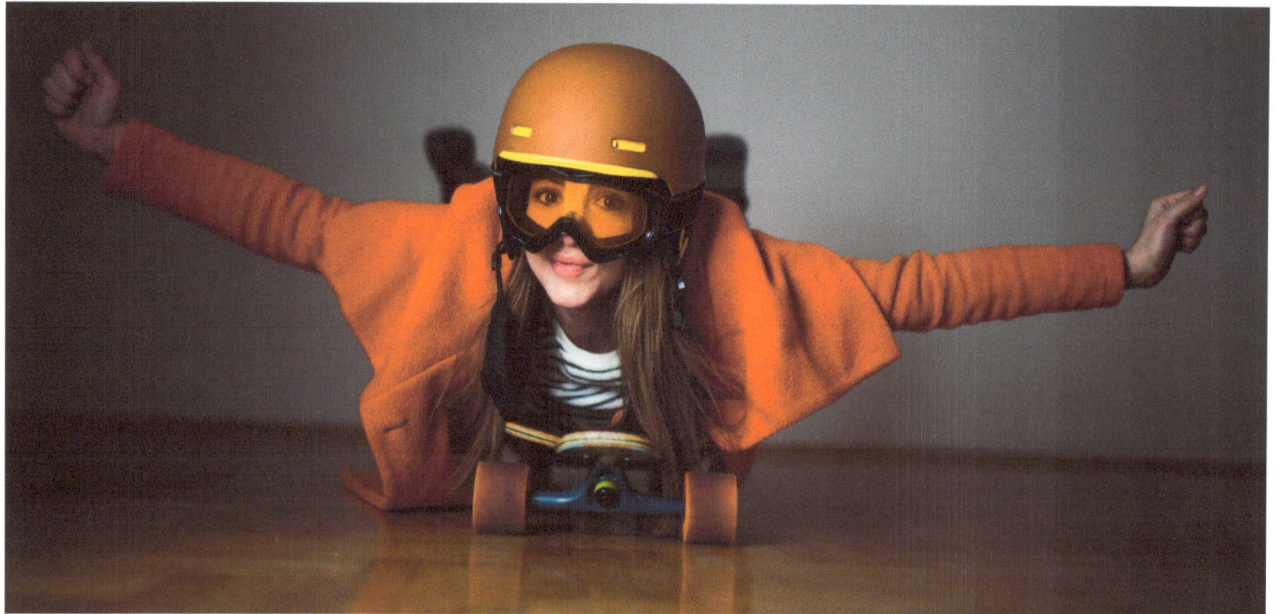

Tools for creative visualisation

Vision boards for big picture visualisation

An easy and fun way to incorporate visualisation into your life is by creating vision boards. Used by entrepreneurs, celebrities, Olympic athletes, and high achievers in every field, vision boards help you to keep your goals and dreams in mind at all times. They give you a clear vision of where you're going and exactly what your life will look like when you've achieved your goals. This is powerful stuff because having this reminder in place helps guide the choices you make each day.

We mentioned before that your brain works tirelessly to achieve the affirmations and images of the goals that you program into your subconscious. With your vision board reminding you of your goals, your brain will prompt you to make choices that get you closer to achieving them.

For example, when you're acting on autopilot, you might grab a bag of chips and head to the chill out in front of the TV until bedtime. But with your vision board at hand, you'll be reminded of your goal to win the title at your upcoming bikini model comp. So, you're more likely to grab your towel and hit the gym.

Creating your vision board can be a lot of fun. If you're into arts and crafts you could make a physical vision board using coloured pens, paper, cardboard, magazines, photos, and whatever else you have in your craft box. If you prefer a digital approach, there are several apps available that will guide you through the process of setting up a virtual vision board.

What goes onto a vision board?

There are no fixed rules regarding how to create your vision board. You're free to make yours in any way you want to. The most important thing to bear in mind when creating your vision board is that, in order to be effective, it needs to be very clear and contain as much detail as possible about the things you want to accomplish. This will ensure that your subconscious mind gets the right message.

Be sure to include photos, pictures, and other items that inspire and motivate you to bring your goals to life. But be careful not to over-clutter it. Having different vision boards for different types of goals (e.g., personal growth, relationships, career, health, social life, finances, education, travel) is a great way to reduce clutter and keep things clear. You could even have one central vision board that covers your top-level goals in all areas and then have smaller boards for specific events, goals or areas in your life, such as your wedding day or overseas trip. Having a career-specific board at your desk is a good way to keep yourself on track at work.

When choosing pictures to include in your vision boards, try to be as specific as possible. For example, if your goal is to purchase a particular car, include pictures of the exact make and model of the car you want.

It's also important to add pictures that show how you will feel when you achieve your goals. You could also use trinkets and/or symbols that have meaning to you to help spark those emotions. Adding a memento (ticket stub, menu, program, coaster, feather, stone) from an event, trip or experience you enjoyed will help you to feel energised and motivated.

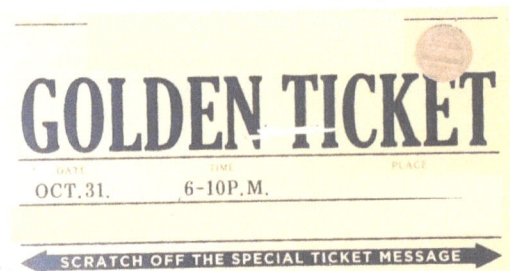

GOLDEN TICKET

OCT. 31.   6-10 P.M.

SCRATCH OFF THE SPECIAL TICKET MESSAGE

Pick objects that remind you of good times and good vibes. Things that, when you look at them, make you feel upbeat and ready to go out there and smash some goals.

You could even add medals, ribbons, invitations or photos from past events, such as a running event or a bikini, bodybuilding or boxing comp, which you want to repeat in future.

Include your affirmations and add motivational quotes, inspirational note cards, and kind words from people who matter to you, such as friends, family or clients. These will encourage you and keep you strong when the going gets tough.

Leave a little space on your vision board where you can add new goals and any inspirational photos or quotes you come across.

You can refresh your vision board as often as you like and make more vision boards as you go along. Once a year, do a complete revamp, keeping those goals that you want to carry over into the new cycle and removing those that have served their purpose.

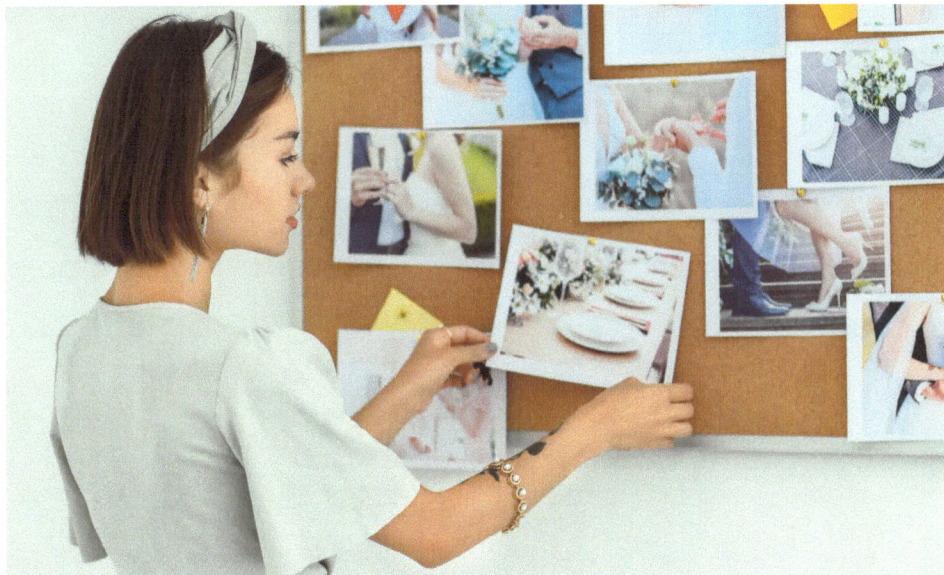

How to create a vision board

1. An A1 or A2 sheet of poster board or cork board

2. Scissors, tape, glue, pins

3. Ribbons, stickers, coloured markers, any other funky decorative stuff

4. Magazines to cut images and quotes from

5. Photos, inspirational quote cards, reminders/souvenirs from places you've been to, postcards from friends, anything you find inspiring that relates to your goals

6. Time to relax and put your board together.

How to create your board:

1. Set aside at least an hour to create your board. Turn off all distractions, clear your space, and put on some relaxing music. You may even want to light a candle, get comfortable, and take 10 deep breaths before you begin to get yourself into a relaxed state of mind.

2. Think about and write down your goals and aspirations for each area of your life. You don't have to cover them all, you can choose one or two to begin with or create a different themed board for each of your goals or events.

3. Write down what you want to achieve, who you want to be, how you want to feel, and whatever inspirational quotes you think will help to keep you motivated.

4. Browse through your collection of magazines, photos, and other items to find the things that best represent your desired goals, emotions, and aspirations.

5. Choose your favourite items and try a few different layouts before you glue or pin them down. Leave a little white space between items to prevent clutter and provide room to add new goals.

Self-hypnosis for daily visualisation

Self-hypnosis is another valuable tool that you can use to unlock the power of creative visualisation. During hypnosis, your brain enters into a highly relaxed and receptive state that helps you to visualise more effectively. Self-hypnosis can be used as part of your daily visualisation process to maximise results. To demonstrate how this works, let's take a detailed look at exactly how you can use self-hypnosis to visualise your goals.

How to use self-hypnosis for creative visualisation

Step 1 Remove distractions and get comfortable

- Choose a favourite secluded spot where you will remain undisturbed by people and devices.

- Wear loose-fitting clothing that won't itch, squeeze, scratch or otherwise distract you.

- Choose something to focus on, or place simple object in your line of sight and focus on that. It could be a coloured bead, a candle flame, a gemstone, a flower or a carved figure. It's up to you.

- You can visualise in silence or with some light instrumental music playing quietly.

- Get comfortable. The recommended posture (which will help to ensure that you don't doze off) is to sit up tall and straight in a comfortable position – either on a chair or on the floor.

Step 2 Decide on your goal for the self-hypnosis session

Settle your mind on what you would like to achieve with this session. For instance, your goal might be to successfully complete today's workout.

Step 3 Focus your gaze on your chosen object

Allow your gaze to fall softly on your chosen focus object.

Step 4 Become conscious of your breath

Begin breathing slowly and deeply – in through your nose and out through your mouth. Imagine that with each exhale your eyelids are becoming heavier.

Step 5 Relax

Continue breathing slowly and deeply until your eyelids feel too heavy to open. Allow your eyes to close and continue to relax even more while focusing only on your slow, steady breath.

Whenever you find your thoughts drifting off on a tangent, simply bring your attention back to your breath.

Step 6 Mentally scan your body

Do a mental scan of your body starting at the crown of your head and slowly working your way down to the soles of your feet. If there is any tension anywhere in the body, imagine exhaling that tension, releasing it, and relaxing even deeper.

Step 7 Visualise

- Start by engaging all your senses to create a peaceful environment.

- Imagine you are surrounded by your favourite colours or you're walking in a cool forest or along a beautiful, secluded beach. Wherever your happy place might be, picture yourself there.

- Add aspects of taste, smell, touch, and sound. Hear the ocean, feel the breeze on your skin, inhale the sweet scent of frangipanis and coconut oil, and taste a delicious juicy mango.

- The deeper you go into this scene, the more relaxed you'll feel. Your body begins to feel very heavy, as though you're about to fall asleep.

- Repeat a mantra, such as 'I am calm' or 'I am at peace', to affirm your relaxed state.

Step 8 Activate your vision

Now you're ready to use visualisation to focus on your goal. Be as specific as possible, use as much detail as you can, and imagine succeeding in whatever steps you need to take to get to your goal. Use all your senses. Try to see, feel, hear, touch, taste, smell, and experience the emotions surrounding your vision. The more vivid you make it, the more your brain will be attracted to it and the stronger your motivation will be to take the steps you need to succeed.

If your goal is to improve the quality of your sleep at night, visualise yourself tucked up in a comfy bed with a light breeze keeping you cool and comfortable. The room is quiet, and you're safe and sound with nothing to do, and no one to demand anything of you. You're free to just let go and enjoy a peaceful night's sleep. Feel the softness of the pillow against your cheek and smell the wonderful aroma of soft soaking rain as you drift towards sleep.

Affirm your vision by projecting feelings of compassion and encouragement towards yourself while mentally repeating your mantra, 'I am sleeping peacefully throughout the night.'

Step 9 Return to normal

When you've completed your visualisation, prepare to leave the hypnotic state by slowly drawing energy back into your body from the world around you. With each inhalation, you draw in positive energy, while with each exhalation, you send that energy flowing through your body. With each breath, you're feeling lighter and more aware of the room around you.

Begin counting slowly down from 10, while mentally affirming that when you reach one you will be energised, your eyes will open, and you will be alert and ready for the day.

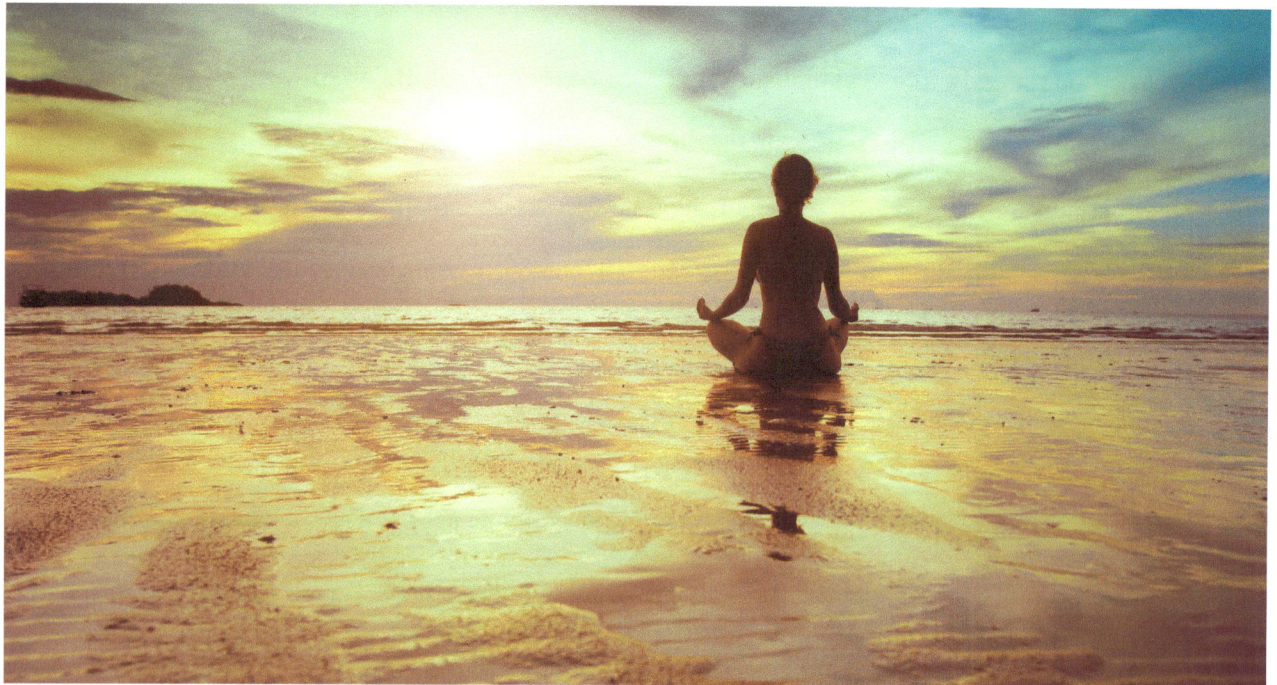

Supercharge yourself for success

By building this simple practice into your daily routine, you will be supercharging your mind and body for success. Your life will begin to align with your vision. You'll feel more inspired, motivated and ready do take the steps needed to create the life you've always dreamed of. What's more, when your motivation flags and inspiration eludes you, you'll have the tools to renew your mindset and program your mighty subconscious for success.

NOTES

4 STEPS TO EFFECTIVE GOAL SETTING

1 KNOW WHERE YOU'RE STARTING FROM

2 KNOW WHERE YOU'RE HEADED

3 KNOW HOW YOU'RE GOING TO GET THERE

4 KNOW WHAT YOU'RE GOING TO DO WHEN THINGS GO WRONG

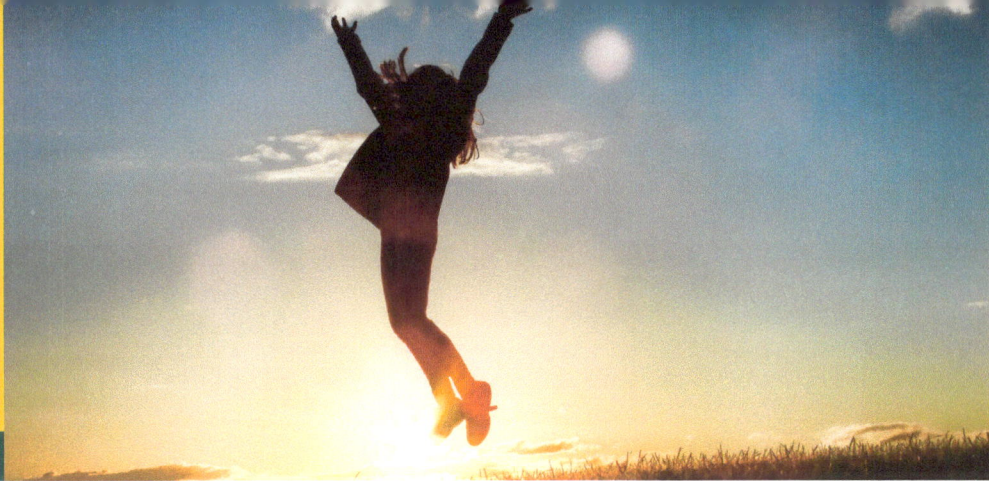

Goal setting

You are never too old to set another goal or to dream a new dream.

C.S. Lewis

In this chapter, we'll provide you with practical strategies for setting goals and cultivating the mental and physical habits you need to succeed. We'll show you how you can set, stick to and smash your goals, and create a life you will love. We're excited about what you're going to achieve, and we're sure you are too. So, let's dive right in.

Four steps to great goal setting

Step 1 Know where you're starting from

Whenever you're planning a journey, the first thing you need to do is be clear about where you're starting from. Your health and wellness journey is no different. This is why we'd like you to be brave and do a quick assessment of where you are right now.

For those of you chasing weight loss, health and fitness goals, this is a great time to start taking some basic measurements, weighing yourself and doing a simple fitness test. Check out the Wellness and Fitness Assessments included at the end of this chapter.

We also highly recommend taking a starting photo of yourself at this point. This is strictly for your eyes only. You don't need to share it with anyone, but *do* take one. You'll thank yourself later. This photo will give you a visual comparison against which you can measure your progress. You'll be amazed by the changes.

We understand that completing this assessment might be incredibly difficult for some people. Coming face-to-face with your current situation can be more than a little confronting. But we want to encourage you to be brave, honest, and, above all, be kind to yourself as you work through the assessments. Importantly, there is no judgement in this. You are simply observing and setting up a benchmark that you can draw on for motivation and inspiration to help you move forward in a new and positive direction.

Remember, you're not defined by who you are now, you're a living, growing, constantly evolving being with the power and the means to change your life whenever you're ready.

You may not be able to go back and make a new start, but you can start right now and make a brand-new ending.

James Sherman

Step 2 Know where you're headed

In this step, you're going to get very clear on where you're headed. It's time to dig deep and decide what you're aiming for.

Think about your overarching goals...

- What is your ultimate goal in following this (or any) program?

- What is the one big goal you've been longing to achieve? Is it to lose weight? Run a marathon? Win a bodybuilding or bikini competition? Become a champion boxer? Or, do you simply want to feel happier and more confident in your own skin?

Don't be afraid to pick the big goals that you've always wanted to achieve, but you've been too afraid to try – until now. It will take just as much effort to change your habits and shoot for a lower target as it will if you were to go for gold, so why not aim high?

What's more, aiming for a goal that stretches you a little makes the journey more exciting. So, be brave and go for that big goal – even if it scares you a bit.

Use your affirmations and visualisations to let go of negativity and limiting beliefs and stay motivated by visualising your success.

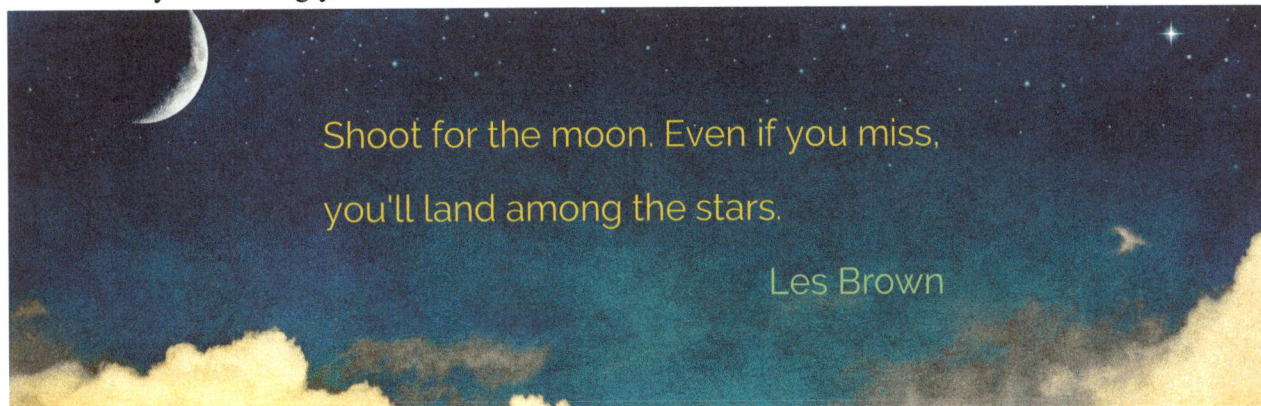

Shoot for the moon. Even if you miss, you'll land among the stars.

Les Brown

Key ingredients of a great big scary goal

It must be deeply personal

Only you can decide on what success looks like for you. Whether it's winning that body-building comp, finishing a marathon, getting down to your goal weight or getting your health back on track so you can be there for your kids – your big goal needs to be deeply personal. And it must be entirely your own.

Remember, there's no right or wrong here, this is your journey. You're in charge of where you're headed. But you must be clear on your desires and your reasons for taking the journey.

It must be passion-driven by a personal why

It's nearly impossible to do what it takes to achieve a big goal if you're not passionate about smashing it. In other words, if your goal is not motivated by a deep, heartfelt desire to succeed, you're setting yourself up for failure. It's that simple.

In the past, you may have tried using willpower to keep yourself on track when trying to reach a big goal. How did that work out for you? Not great? Don't worry, you're not alone. And it's not your fault. At some point, we've all tried to achieve our goals using willpower alone and failed miserably. Why? Because willpower is a limited resource.

Imagine you're trying to lose weight. You've decided to use willpower to fend off temptation and stick to your goal. Once you've spent all day avoiding morning teas, politely declining offers of snacks from well-meaning colleagues, and resisting the temptation offered by the numerous convenience stores and vending machines that you pass during your commute, you simply have nothing left in your willpower tank. It's no wonder then that, by the time you get home, you give in and polish off that tub of ice cream.

So, instead of relying on willpower, you need to lean into your why – that is your reason(s) for wanting to succeed at your goal. When you know your why, you'll be better equipped to deal with any temptations and obstacles that get in your way.

When temptation comes around, remind yourself that you're chasing this goal for a reason, and that reason is more important to you than eating that second piece of cake or whatever other goal-sabotaging behaviour you were contemplating.

Another important reason to keep your why at the top of your mind is that, if you forget your why, you'll start seeing your goal as an obligation that has been imposed on you, instead of a choice you have made. Nothing will kill your motivation faster and put you off your goal more effectively than feeling that you're doing it because you *have* to.

Remembering that you chose this goal for a very good reason and reminding yourself of what that reason is (your why) will see you through the tough times when it all seems too hard, and you feel like giving up.

> 66 When you know your "why", you can endure any how.
> John O'Leary (adapted from Friedrich Nietzsche)

The best way to keep ourselves motivated is to take control of our choices and to see them as affirmations of our values. We need to be able to connect our small tasks to our larger aspirations.

Charles Duhig

What Charles Duhigg is saying is...

1. You're in control of achieving your goals through the choices you make.

2. You need to make choices based on what's important to you (i.e., your values) rather than on temporary feelings, cravings, and emotions.

3. Every small action you take (e.g., polishing off the ice cream) makes a difference in whether or not you're going to achieve your goals.

4. You should weigh these small actions up against your why before you decide to take them.

5. Get clear on your why and use it to guide your choices.

6. Make it the lock screen image on your phone. Print it out and stick it on your bathroom mirror, your fridge, the pantry door or your kid's forehead (okay maybe not that, but you get the idea).

7. Do whatever you can to remind yourself of your why at every opportunity.

8. Make sure your daily actions (no matter how small) are guided by your why.

It must be perfectly clear and specific

If you've been spinning around on the hamster wheel of life, always wishing for, but never quite hitting your goals, this step might make all the difference for you.

You see, to be effective, your goal must be very clear and specific, meaning you need to do more than say 'I want to be healthier' or 'I want to lose weight.'

You need to get down to the nitty-gritty and decide exactly what that means *for you*. Perhaps, your big scary goal is to get into the best shape of your life. You need to refine your objective, so you're clear on exactly what you're aiming for.

You may already be aware of the SMART goal system for creating goals. It's really handy for nailing down the kind of clear and specific goals we're talking about.

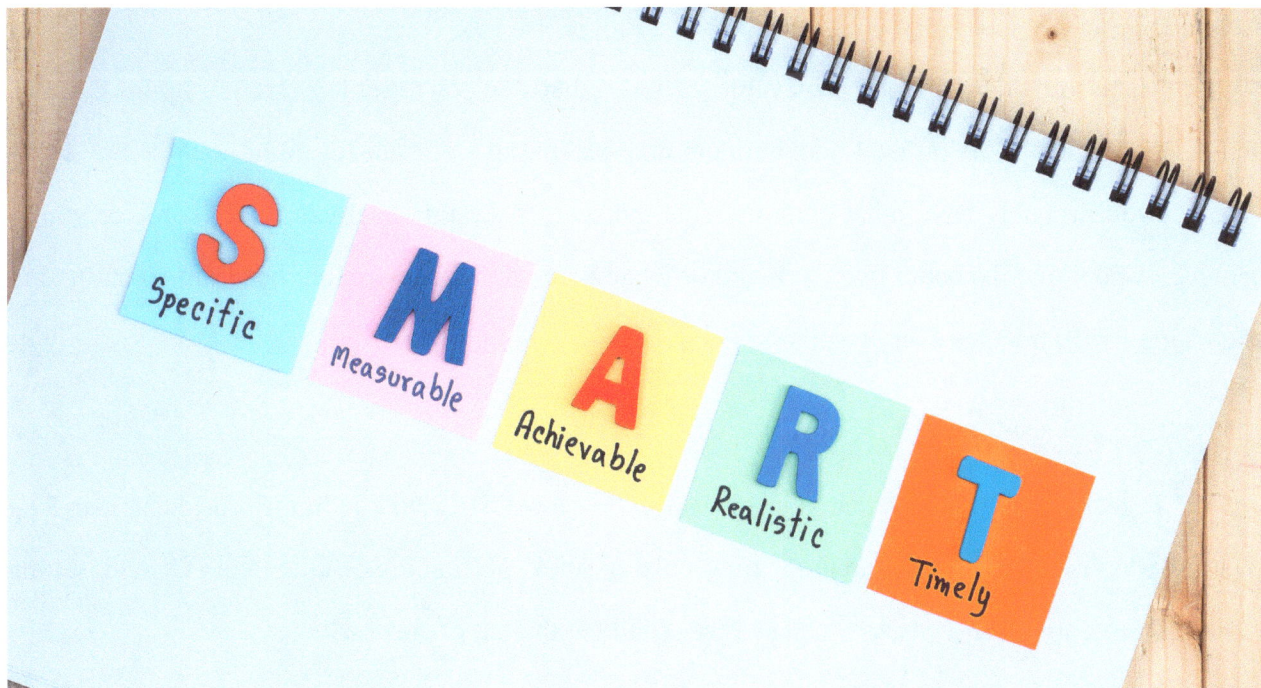

To be SMART, your goal needs to be

Specific

Add as much detail to your goal as possible. So, instead of saying 'I want to lose weight' try saying 'I am committed to losing 5 kg.'

Measurable

Make sure that your goal is measurable, so you can see your progress and know when you've achieved success. For example, instead of saying 'I want to eat more fruit.' You could say 'I am committed to eating two serves of fruit per day.'

Achievable

Make sure your goals are achievable *for you*, otherwise you're setting yourself up for failure and disappointment. Professional bodybuilders may be able to work out for eight hours a day, every day, but you probably have other commitments that will make this goal extremely hard for you to achieve. A goal that fits better into the realm of what is possible for you might be, 'I am committed to exercising for 30 minutes every morning.'

Realistic

It goes without saying, that your goals need to be realistic. No one in the world can lose 5 kg overnight or run their first marathon after only a week of training. Being realistic and setting manageable goals make it easier to achieve them and get that hit of success.

For example, if your big scary goal is to run your first marathon, but you're not a runner yet, then break that sucker down and say 'I want to be able to run 100 m without stopping by the end of the week.' If you want to lose 5 kg in five weeks, set yourself the goal of losing 100 g per day.

Time-based

Saying you want to run a marathon without giving yourself a time frame is just wishful thinking. And no one ever achieved anything just by wishful thinking.

Think back to high school for a minute. When did you finally get down to studying for that test or writing that essay? If you were like most of us, it was probably just before the deadline.

If they'd told you that you could hand your essay in whenever you felt like it? You'd probably keep putting it off indefinitely. Right?

It's the same with achieving your goals – you must have a deadline. And, just like back at school, you can't put things off until the day before the deadline and expect to get good results. You've got to set your deadline, claim your target, and hustle all the way to the finish line.

To summarise, an example of a SMART goal would be

I am committed to running 5 km without stopping in 7 weeks' time, starting today.

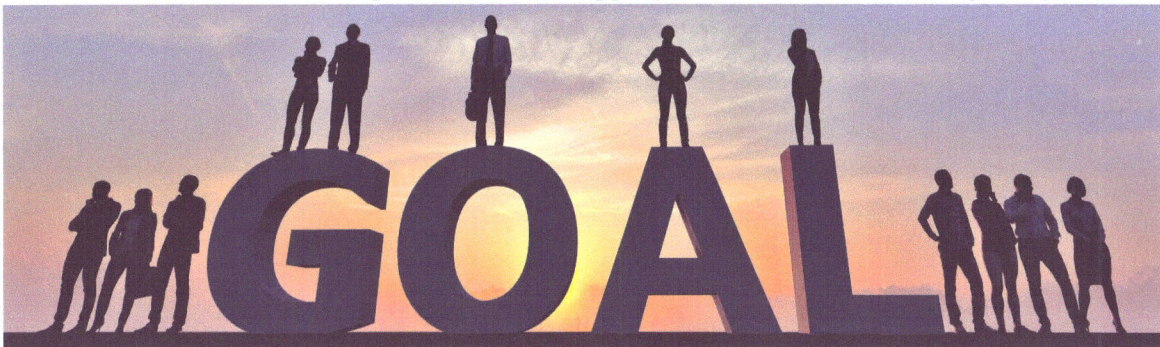

Step 3 Know how you're going to get there

Like so much else in life, achieving a healthy mind and body requires more than just a desire for change. You need to take action. And, as we mentioned earlier, those actions need to be aligned with your big goal and driven by your why.

The best way to approach this is to take that big scary goal and break it down into series of steps that are easy to take. These steps will form the basis of the plan that will ultimately lead to you smashing your goal.

> **"** A goal without a plan is just a wish.
>
> Antoine de Saint-Exupéry

Questions to ask when formulating your plan:

- What steps are you going to take over the next few days, weeks or months to make your goal a reality?

- How much time will you need each day to make this happen? Will you set aside 30 minutes each day or block out a few days a week to work on your goals?

- What resources or supplies will you need to invest in?

- How much are you willing or able to spend to make this dream a reality? Draw up a budget.

- What research/resources do you need before you begin? For example, websites, books or courses.

- Do you need an accountability partner, trainer, mentor, training buddy, and/or life coach?

- Are there groups you could join to help keep you motivated?

Taking our SMART goal example of being able to run 5 km without stopping in seven weeks' time, your smaller goals might look something like this.

Before Day 1, gather the resources you need to achieve your goal:

- Find a "couch-to-5 km" running program – there are plenty of free ones online or you could find one in a book or magazine or ask a running coach or personal trainer to provide you with one.

- Find a strength training program for runners – there are plenty of free ones online or you could find one in a book or magazine, hire a personal trainer or join a gym, Pilates or yoga studio.

- Commit to researching, planning, preparing, and following your nutrition plan. We'll look more closely at nutrition later in the book, but for now, take a look at the various nutrition apps available – some of which provide excellent free resources that allow you to research, plan, and record your nutrition.

- Block off 30 minutes per day, three times per week for running training, and commit to following your "couch-to-5 km" running program.

- Commit to doing 30 minutes of strength training (e.g., swimming, yoga, aerobics, a gym workout or a training video workout) twice per week on days when you're not running.

- Commit to at least one rest day per week to give your muscles a chance to recover.

- Get kitted out with the right running shoes, socks, sunscreen, hat, and moisture-wicking clothing. Optional extras include smartwatches, smartphones, portable media players, and headphones.

- Find an accountability buddy, running coach or training partner or join a running or walking group in your area.

- For extra motivation, try to find and sign up for a 5 km fun run event that's approximately seven weeks away. You could even use this as an opportunity to raise funds for your favourite charity.

From Day 1 onwards:

- Follow your training plan (including your rest days). No excuses. No exceptions.
- Eat three healthy meals and two healthy snacks per day.
- Stay hydrated by drinking eight glasses (approximately two litres) of water per day.
- Get at least eight hours of sleep each night.

Step 4 Know what to do when things go wrong

Once you're crystal clear about what you have to do to get where you want to go, it's time to consider how you're going to handle setbacks and obstacles.

It's easy to get caught up in the excitement of goal setting. But, ask anyone who has made New Year's resolutions on the first of January only to toss them out the window by the first of February, and they'll tell you that life tends to throw curveballs at you – just when you think it's going to be all plain sailing.

If you're not prepared for these, you could be left feeling despondent and ready to give up on your dreams in a very short time. So, we're going to be proactive and take some time here to work out responses to the challenges you're likely to face when trying to change your life and achieve your goals. The challenges that hamper your progress usually fall into three broad categories: internal challenges, external challenges within your control, and external challenges outside of your control. Let's take a look at some examples.

Internal challenges

These challenges are the mental arguments and battles you fight against your worst enemy and greatest ally – yourself. They include all your limiting beliefs, excuses, and negative thoughts that sound like legitimate reasons at the time.

Things you hear yourself saying, day in and day out, such as:

- I can't.
- I'm too tired.
- I haven't got any time.
- I just don't feel like it.
- I'm just not motivated.
- I'll do it tomorrow.
- I'm too unfit at the moment.
- I'll wait until I've lost some weight.
- I've had a bad day, so I deserve to eat that box of donuts.
- I'll start over again on Monday.

It's important to see these for what they really are – your mind playing tricks on you. As long as you allow them to, these negative thoughts and limiting beliefs will throw obstacles of doubt and misery into your path, paralysing you and preventing you from moving forward towards your goal.

Fortunately, you can use the visualisation and affirmation techniques you learnt in the previous chapters to overcome your internal challenges and move forward. Here's how.

How to overcome a lack of motivation

When you're feeling unmotivated and just thinking about working out brings out your sulky inner child, it's time to remind yourself of your why. Remember, you're not doing this to punish your inner child or to impress anyone else, you're doing this for a very personal, very meaningful reason. Try to focus on that reason and encourage the sulky inner child to help you achieve your goal.

Just like willpower, motivation is never there when you need it. So, don't waste time waiting around for it. Go out and smash some goals instead.

Consistency is the key to getting where you want to go, so use your affirmations and visualisation techniques to stay on track. By repeating your affirmations out loud with feeling, looking at your vision board, and/or combining visualisation with self-hypnosis, you'll be reminded in a powerful way of your reasons for wanting to achieve your goals. You'll be able to overcome the feelings of despondency and be inspired to do what it takes to achieve your dreams.

Not enough time?

What if you don't have enough time to pursue your dreams? If this is something you struggle with, try reframing this thought with the realisation that we all get the same 24 hours every day – no more, no less. It's how you spend that time that matters.

It's always going to be easier to live the same life you're living now, saying that you don't have the time to chase your dreams, and never achieving your desired goals.

But, if you tenderly care for the hours you have, you'll find the time to do the daily things you need to do that will get you closer to your goals.

Here's a simple time-tracking exercise you can do to help you find the time you need:

- Grab a piece of paper, use the space provided or open a spreadsheet.
- Starting from the time you usually wake up in the morning, jot down the time in 15-minute intervals to form a column on the right-hand side of the page.
- In the adjacent column, record your activities during each 15-minute interval.
- Repeat for all seven days of the week.

At the end of the week, review your activities:

- Are there any areas where you could find 15 or even 30 minutes to spend on something that will get you closer to your goal?
- Could you use your lunch break more constructively?
- Perhaps, you could sacrifice half an hour of TV each night?
- Or maybe you could set the alarm half an hour earlier and tackle your goal-oriented tasks first thing in the morning?

If, after doing this exercise, you're still struggling to find time to work on your goal, it's possible that you're overcommitted, in which case, you could be at risk of burnout. It may be time to dial things back a bit.

Take a moment to think about what's really important to you and prioritise those things. Then delegate or abdicate from the less important things that are demanding your time. If you feel unable do this on your own, reach out to a life coach or counsellor for help.

TIME TRACKER

Time	Activity	DATE:
		DAY:

Believe. Train. Nourish. Achieve.

External challenges within your control

This includes life events, such as a heavier-than-normal workload, the weather (when it's too hot/cold/wet), your finances, and the availability of trainers or training partners. Just like your negative thoughts and limiting beliefs, these things can seem like legitimate reasons to delay taking action, but they can easily be reframed so that you can get on with achieving your goals.

Wait, are you saying the weather is under my control?

Um, no. But this is what we mean by reframing. The weather is not under your control, but how you respond to it is. When it comes to training, for example, it may be too hot/cold/wet to go out for a run, but there are other options, right? Instead of saying 'Oh dear, the weather's too hot, so I can't do my run today.' You could reframe the situation by saying 'Well, the weather's too hot for me to run outdoors, but I really want to stay on track with my program, so I'll go to the gym and run on the treadmill instead.' Or you could wait until it's cooler and go running in the evening with a running group or a training buddy. Alternatively, you could do a home workout instead of going for a run.

The important thing is to adapt your actions to the circumstances and stay focused on achieving your goal.

What about finances? Surely, that's not always under my control?

We are all at the mercy of the economy, and our personal circumstances differ vastly, but here again, there are options available. If finances are a concern, and your goal is to get fit, you could try walking or running for exercise, instead of costly gym memberships. If running's not for you, there are plenty of free workout videos or printouts available online that can be done in the comfort of your own home. Failing that, you could pay a visit to your local library, take out a book on exercise for free and get started in your living room.

Surely, I can't help it if my trainer/training partner is out of action?

When your trainer or training buddy's out of action, it can be tempting to stop training and wait until they recover. But that's not getting you any closer to your goal.

Instead of giving up, see it as an opportunity to keep on training on your own. You could reframe this by thinking, 'This is my chance to prove to myself that I can do it on my own. I'm going to get out there and smash it.'

Forget it, I'm already feeling overwhelmed by all my commitments

With work, family, kids, and community to juggle, it can be hard to see where goal-oriented activities fit into your already packed-to-the-rafters life.

As mentioned before during our time-tracking exercise, you can start by identifying and reducing or eliminating those things in your daily life that are neither urgent nor important. For example, if you reduce or, better yet, kick the nightly TV habit, you'll be amazed at how much extra time you have.

You can also save energy and reduce decision fatigue by automating or delegating as much of your life as possible. For example, you could set up automated bill payments online and/or assign chores and responsibilities to family members instead of trying to do it all yourself. This not only saves time but also encourages teamwork within the family. Plus, the kids will learn new life skills.

Another approach is to start by asking 'What is the one thing I can do each day that will get me closer to my goal?' It may be as simple as taking half an hour to exercise every morning.

Block out the time needed for your daily goal-oriented task before adding anything else to your schedule. We recommend setting aside early mornings for goal-oriented tasks, such as running, working out or practising. You'll be better able to stay focused on your goal if it's the first thing you tackle every day. And, by getting your goal-related tasks out of the way in the morning, they're done and dusted for the day. No matter what the rest of the day throws at you, you've taken care of the important stuff that will get you closer to the life you long for.

External challenges beyond your control

These are tougher obstacles and events that strike without warning, such as a sick child, car accident or family crisis. You clearly have no control over these. They need to be dealt with and often sap your energy, making it difficult to put in the time and effort you need to chase your goals.

Sometimes, exercise, yoga, meditation, and other lifestyle goal-oriented activities can offer a lifeline in the midst of crisis – a 30-minute respite from the trauma of life.

At other times, your external challenges might derail your journey completely. If this happens, try not to stress out about it. Just make sure that, once the issue is resolved, you dive back into your plan and pick up where you left off. Or, if that's not possible, restart the process from scratch, creating new goals that are better suited to your altered circumstances.

GOAL SETTING CHEAT SHEET

Pick out five big goals

- Make sure your big goals are SMART.

- Think about why you want to achieve these goals.

- Write down your why, print it out and put it where you'll see it.

- Break down each big goal into smaller achievable SMART goals.

- Define the daily thing(s) you need to do to get closer to your goal.

- Create a daily schedule that prioritises your goal-related tasks.

Identify internal challenges

- Write down as many internal challenges you can think of that might hinder you from achieving your goal.

- Reframe your responses to show how you will overcome these.

Identify external challenges within your control

- Write down as many external challenges under your control as you can think of that might hinder you from achieving your goal.

- Reframe your responses to show how you will overcome these.

Identify external challenges beyond your control

- Write down as many external challenges beyond your control as you can think of that might hinder you from achieving your goal.

- If possible, reframe your responses to show how you might overcome these or consider ways you could use your affirmations, meditation, mindfulness, creative visualisation, self-hypnosis – and even your goal-related action steps – as a lifeline to help you through the tough times.

MY GOAL IS...

WHY IS THIS GOAL IMPORTANT TO ME?

STEPS TO TAKE

- [ ]
- [ ]
- [ ]
- [ ]
- [ ]

CHALLENGES	RESPONSES

DEADLINE _____   MARK AS COMPLETE ☐

DAILY PLANNER

DATE: _____

DAY: _____

TO DO LIST:

☐ _____

☐ _____

☐ _____

☐ _____

☐ _____

☐ _____

☐ _____

☐ _____

☐ _____

☐ _____

NOTES:

_____

_____

_____

_____

_____

6:00 AM

6:30 AM

7:00 AM

7:30 AM

8:00 AM

8:30 AM

9:00 AM

9:30 AM

10:00 AM

10:30 AM

11:00 AM

11:30 AM

12:00 PM

12:30 PM

1:00 PM

1:30 PM

2:00 PM

2:30 PM

3:00 PM

3:30 PM

4:00 PM

4:30 PM

5:00 PM

Believe. Train. Nourish. Achieve.

WEEKLY PLANNER

MONDAY
Date

GOALS	ACTIONS	REWARDS
_____	_____	_____
_____	_____	_____
_____	_____	_____
_____	_____	_____

TUESDAY
Date

GOALS	ACTIONS	REWARDS
_____	_____	_____
_____	_____	_____
_____	_____	_____
_____	_____	_____

WEDNESDAY
Date

GOALS	ACTIONS	REWARDS
_____	_____	_____
_____	_____	_____
_____	_____	_____
_____	_____	_____

THURSDAY
Date

GOALS	ACTIONS	REWARDS
_____	_____	_____
_____	_____	_____
_____	_____	_____
_____	_____	_____

FRIDAY
Date

GOALS	ACTIONS	REWARDS
_____	_____	_____
_____	_____	_____
_____	_____	_____
_____	_____	_____

FOUR WEEKS AT-A-GLANCE

	WEEK 1	WEEK 2	WEEK 3	WEEK 4
MON				
TUE				
WED				
THU				
FRI				

Believe. Train. Nourish. Achieve.

WELLNESS ASSESSMENT

START DATE:

WEEK	START				
WEIGHT*					
BMI**					
CHEST /cm Across nipples					
WAIST /cm At belly button					
THIGH /cm At widest point					
BICEP/cm At widest point					

* Hop on the scale first thing in the morning, after going to the toilet and before eating or drinking anything.

**BMI (Body Mass Index) is calculated by dividing your weight (kg) by your height (m); then dividing the result by your height (m) again.

FITNESS ASSESSMENT

WEEK	START				
Time to jog/ run/ walk 1 km					
Sit-ups in 1 minute					
Wall-sit max time min + sec*					
Plank max time min + sec **					
Sit & reach /cm ***					

* Stand with your back against the wall, feet hip-width apart. Slide your back down the wall until your knees are bent at 90° as if you are sitting on an invisible stool. Hold the position for as long as you can. Record your time.

** Sit on your mat with your legs straight in front of you. Extend your torso and arms along your legs reaching towards your toes. Measure the distance from fingertips to toes.

*** Lie on your stomach on the mat. Resting on your elbows and toes, lift your torso and legs off the ground. Keep your back straight, and your head, neck, and bottom in line with your spine. Hold the position for as long as you can.

Before attempting this assessment, please consult a fitness professional for advice on how to complete the exercises safely.

Train

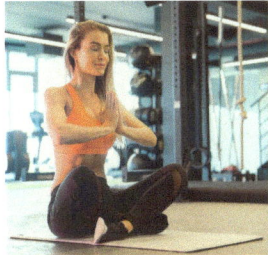

Mindful training

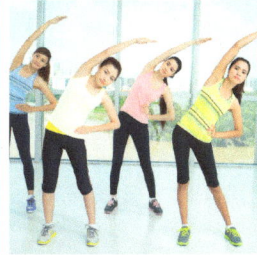

Warming up

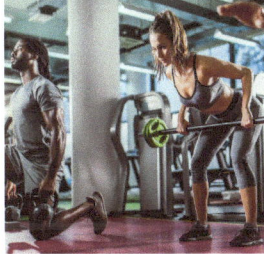

Training
&
Getting back
to fitness

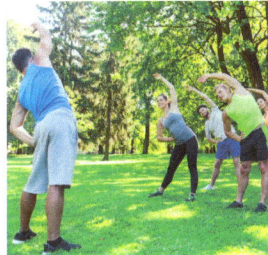

Cooling down
&
Rest & sleep

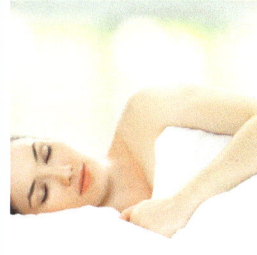

"Nothing happens until something moves.
Albert Einstein

Your goals are set. Your why is stuck to the fridge door. Your wellness and fitness assessments are done and dusted. You've got a great program and a pile of strategies to handle setbacks. You're ready for change. But nothing's going to happen if you don't take action and make it happen.

It's time to get out there and get moving.

There are so many different training approaches, methods, and activities, that it's impossible to cover them all in one book – let alone one section of a book. And the intensity, structure, frequency, and duration of your training program will vary depending on your own unique fitness level, abilities, and goals. So, to give you as much value as possible, we're going to focus on the fundamental principles for success that apply to all training programs and approaches. You'll be able to apply these principles to your training program to ensure you get the most out of your workouts.

We'll explain how to use mindfulness to get the best results from your warm-up, training, and cool-down sessions and provide practical tips to optimise your training and prevent injury.

We'll also take a look at some of the most popular and effective training methods. Finally, we'll examine the importance of rest and sleep and share ways to get the quality sleep and rest your body needs.

Please consult a healthcare professional before following this advice and/or beginning any training program to ensure that it is right for you.

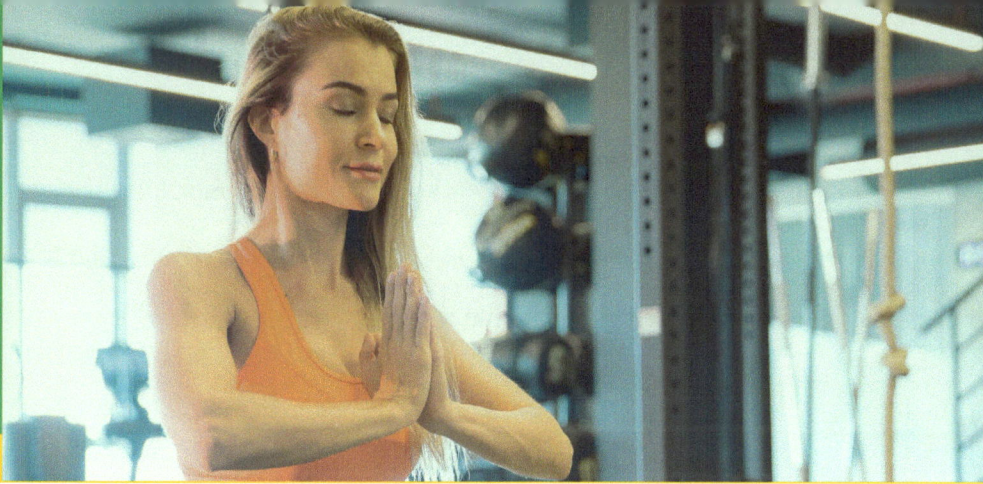

Mindful training

I hated every minute of training. But I said, 'Don't quit.
Suffer now and live the rest of your life as a champion.'
Muhammed Ali

Let's face it, training is hard – even for the greatest athletes among us. It's supposed to be. And because it's challenging, we are often tempted to mentally check out. Our minds wander off, and we start to think about other things while we do our reps. Before we know it, we're no longer focusing on what we're doing, but instead, we're thinking about how good it's going to be to go out on the weekend, how cute the cat is when she sleeps or what we should do about the new puppy who's chewing up all our shoes. This may take our minds off the pain, but it won't help us get the most out of our training.

Research shows that mindful training can dramatically improve results. So, instead of worrying, wondering, and generally zoning out, try being mindful during your training sessions.

You'll recall from the Believe section of this book that mindfulness involves being fully present in each and every moment of life and seeking out the joy in that moment. Applying this principle to your workouts means paying attention to your body, concentrating on what you're doing and how you're doing it and finding joy in each moment of your workout. By being mindful when you work out, you'll actually start enjoying your workouts more. Plus, there are loads of other benefits that come with mindful training. Let's take a closer look at some of them.

The benefits of mindful training

1. Mindful training improves flow

Zoning out and listening to your favourite podcast or playlist is great when it comes to getting through a session of endurance training, such as walking, jogging or running. It puts you into a meditative state and allows your mind to roam while your body does something more or less monotonous.

But, when you become too distracted, and you're not focusing on what you're doing during your workouts, you miss out on the amazing sense of flow and harmony that only comes through mindful training. When you're fully present during your workouts, you'll be tuning in to the feeling of pure joy that comes from seeing your own strength and power in action. Try it; you'll love it.

2. Mindful training improves form

When you rush mindlessly through your training, thinking about the kids, your partner or your job, you're not focusing on your form. As a result, your workouts become less effective, and you run the risk of injury.

By taking things slowly and focusing on form, you're building a mind-muscle connection that improves muscle activation and delivers better results.

What is form?

Simply put, form relates to how you do each exercise.

From start to finish, your form includes:

1. Warming up properly.

2. Focusing on the muscle group you're working on at each moment.

3. Maintaining good posture during the exercise.

4. Breathing properly during the exercise.

5. Cooling down properly.

3. Mindful training improves your mental health

Research shows that adding mindfulness to your workouts and focusing on what you're doing during your training sessions actually reduces stress, depression, and anxiety. Plus, it improves your performance and allows you to sleep better.

4. Mindful training improves your physical health

Mindful exercising has been shown to improve cardiovascular health, including better breathing, heart rate, and parasympathetic activity. Mindful workouts also result in lower BMI and lower fasting blood sugar levels.

5. Mindful training improves your attitude and your lifestyle

Mindful training helps cultivate a more positive attitude towards physical health. This has a snowball effect because your positive attitude spurs you on towards more positive behaviours (e.g., sticking to you training program), which in turn, leads to better physical health and even more healthy lifestyle choices. In fact, people who practice mindfulness have also been shown to feel more satisfied after their workouts and are better able to stick to their training programs.

> **Don't remind yourself how tired and weak you feel. Stay positive. Every rep. Every step. Brings you closer to your goals.**
> Unknown

How to be mindful during training

With all the benefits that mindful training offers, it's worth knowing how to build mindfulness into your daily exercise routine. Here are a few ways you can stay fully present and focused on what you are doing at each moment of your workout.

1. Set intentions for your workout and focus on them

In the chapter on Goal Setting, we talked about breaking your big scary goals down into bite-sized chunks that are easy to achieve. As you approach your daily workout, remind yourself of the mini-goals you set for this workout and focus on those goals while you're doing the exercises.

For example, if your big goal is to run a half-marathon in 20 weeks' time and today is a cross-training session, your mini-goals may include:

A. Doing each exercise in my program with proper form.

B. Completing today's training session to the best of my abilities.

C. Working out with enthusiasm.

D. Giving my all during my HIIT (high-intensity interval training) session.

2. Focus on the muscles involved in each exercise

Instead of watching other people in the gym and comparing yourself to them or thinking about other things during your workout, mindful training helps you to focus on your own body, on the muscles you are using, on what you are experiencing, and on what your instructor is telling you.

When you train mindfully, you will be paying close attention to how your body is positioned before starting the exercise and be mindful of doing each move correctly for maximum effect.

For example, if you're going to do squats, take a moment to check:

- Are your feet between hip- and shoulder-width apart?
- Are your toes pointing slightly outward (between 5°and 15°)?
- Are the tips of your toes in line with each other?
- Is your weight centred on your heels?
- Is your back straight, and your spine neutral?
- Are your shoulders back and relaxed?
- Is your chest open, and your core engaged?

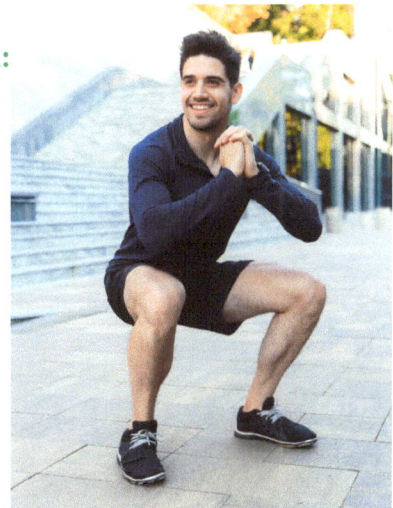

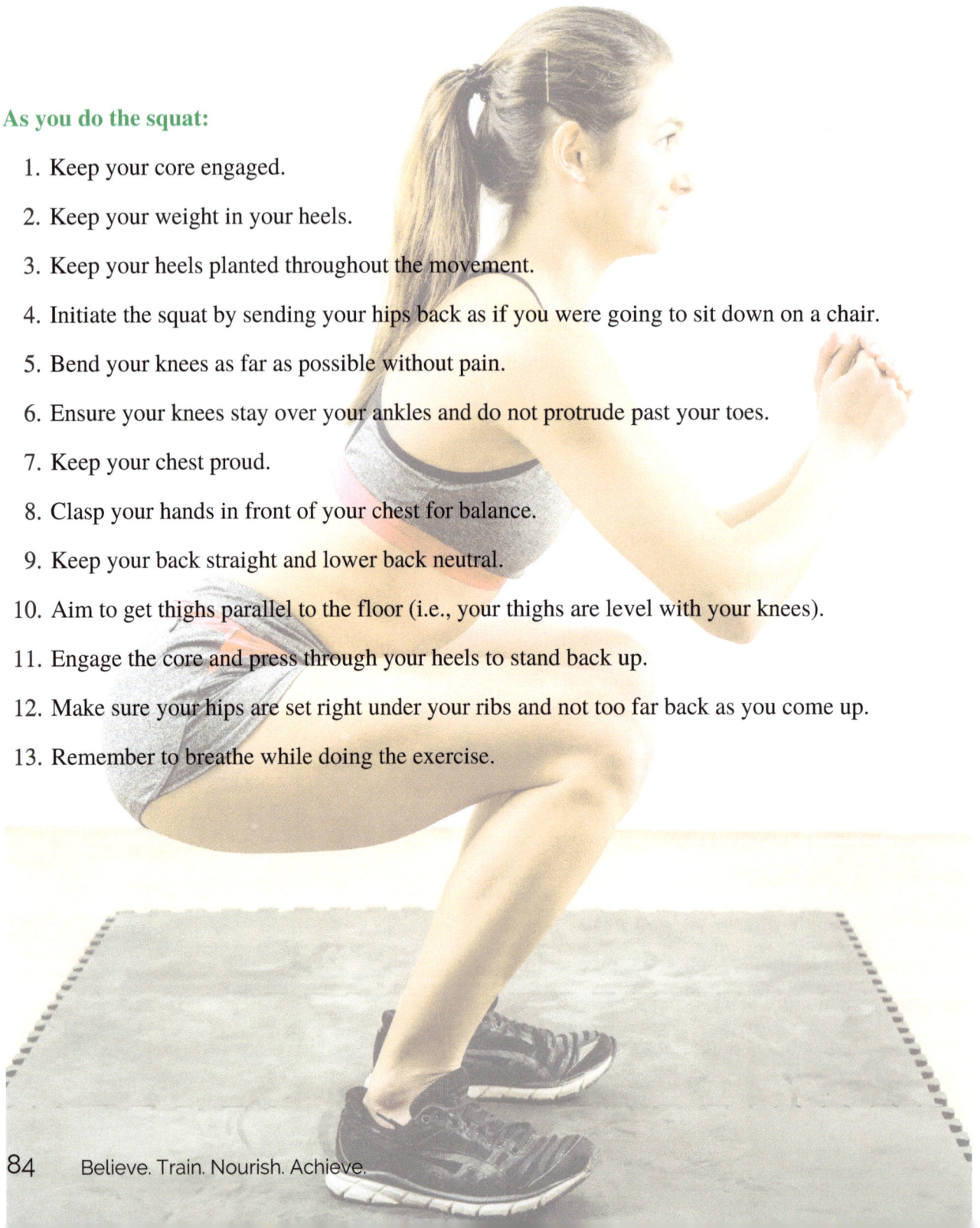

As you do the squat:

1. Keep your core engaged.

2. Keep your weight in your heels.

3. Keep your heels planted throughout the movement.

4. Initiate the squat by sending your hips back as if you were going to sit down on a chair.

5. Bend your knees as far as possible without pain.

6. Ensure your knees stay over your ankles and do not protrude past your toes.

7. Keep your chest proud.

8. Clasp your hands in front of your chest for balance.

9. Keep your back straight and lower back neutral.

10. Aim to get thighs parallel to the floor (i.e., your thighs are level with your knees).

11. Engage the core and press through your heels to stand back up.

12. Make sure your hips are set right under your ribs and not too far back as you come up.

13. Remember to breathe while doing the exercise.

Believe. Train. Nourish. Achieve.

3. Slow down and refocus

Mindful training helps you to slow down and remember your why. If you find that you're rushing through the exercises without putting much effort in, or you're struggling to get through a workout, it's time to take a moment and be more mindful.

Slow down and reflect on why you decided to make exercise a priority in the first place.

Refocus on your intentions for the workout and remember your why. For example:

1. This workout will help me have more energy for my kids.

2. I'm going to feel so much better for having done my workout today.

3. This workout is getting me closer to my goal of running my first half marathon.

4. I deserve to take care of myself, and training is part of that.

5. I'm going to feel more relaxed once I've finished my workout.

4. Let your workout be *your* time

Try reframing your training sessions as time you're dedicating to helping *you* feel better. Think of your workouts as your special time and acknowledge that you deserve this time. Then allow yourself to savour every moment.

Focus on your muscles and feel the strength you're developing. Enjoy the endorphins flowing through your body and the sense of joy and accomplishment you feel after completing each set.

Remember, you can't be there for your loved ones if you don't take the time to care for yourself. So, give yourself permission to take the time to do your workout.

5. Don't forget to breathe

Mindful breathing is an essential part of mindful training. Breathing helps you to relax and destress. Plus, your breath helps you to get energy and oxygen into your muscles as you exercise.

Focusing on your breath is also an excellent way to bring yourself back into the moment. If you find your mind wandering during your workout, simply take a second to concentrate on breathing, and you'll soon be fully present once more.

> " Celebrate your victories no matter how small they may seem. Nobody knows more than you, how much they cost you.
>
> Karla S (K.S) (@proactiveyellowworld)

6. Leave on a high and celebrate your achievements

As you take the time to cool down and stretch after your workout, think about and celebrate all the good things that happened during your training. Appreciate how good your body feels now that you've spent time focusing on it and how good it feels to be fitter and stronger than yesterday.

Before you leave, take a moment to lie quietly and relax completely. This gives you the opportunity to soak up all the benefits of your workout. Think of it as five minutes of delicious me time that you can look forward to during your workout. Having this little rest at the end of each workout will help to motivate you to return for your next session.

Now that you've got the hang of mindful training, it's time to take a look in a little more detail at the ways to get the most out of each of the three stages that make up your typical workout: warming up, training, and cooling down.

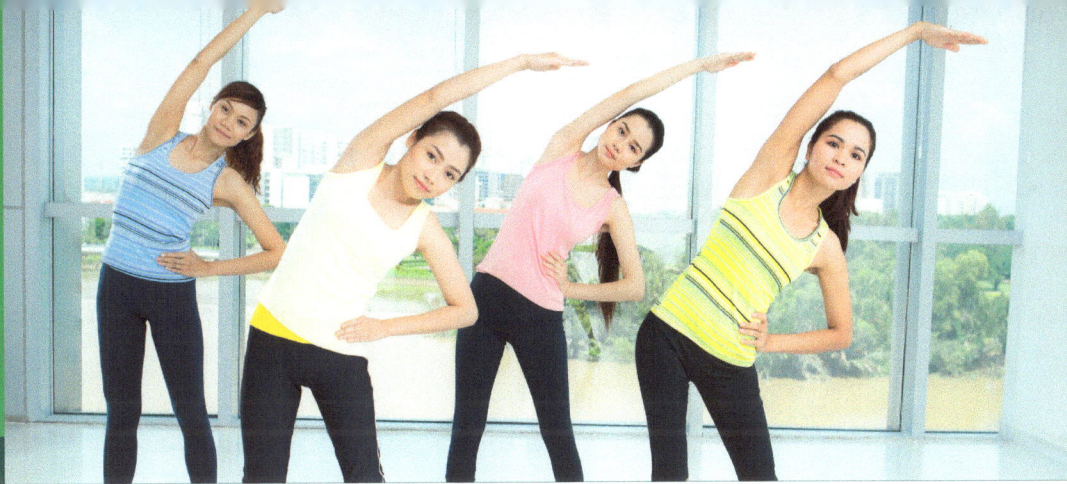

Warming up

I practice every day, I warm up before I play.
Travis Barker

One of our running buddies came over to Australia from England. He turned up to every run fully kitted out in a tracksuit and a beanie cap – no matter what the weather was like. Even in Summer. In Queensland...

When we asked him why he always wore this get-up every time he went for a run, even in the blazing Queensland heat, his answer was surprisingly simple.

'Well,' he said. 'I've worn my tracksuit and beanie on all my runs, ever since I started running years ago back in the UK. Now, whenever I put them on, my body knows that I'm going for a run.'

Your warm-up is a lot like our friend's tracksuit and beanie. It tells your body that you're going to be exercising. And, while we don't recommend running in a tracksuit and beanie in forty-degree heat, we do recommend doing a good warm-up. That's because your warm-up gets the nerve-endings firing, the muscles loosened up, and the whole body ready for the big event.

A good warm-up gives your body the opportunity to ease into the workout by doing exercises at a slower pace and lower intensity. Warming up helps your body prepare for the physical and cardiovascular demands that your workout will place on it. When you take just 5 to10 minutes to warm up properly, you're preparing your cardiovascular system for aerobic activity by raising your body temperature and increasing your heart rate and blood flow to your muscles. This is great for reducing stress on your heart and other muscles. Plus, it helps you get more out of your workout and reduces the risk of injury.

How to warm up properly

For best results, make your warm-up part of your training routine. It goes without saying that you should do your warm-up right before you start your workout. If you leave too much time between the two, all the good work you've done getting your muscles and heart ready to go will be wasted as your body returns to its previous state – cold muscles, lower heart rate, and all.

Focus on warming up the large muscle groups, such as your leg muscles, first. Going for a walk or marching on the spot are great ways to start your warm-up. Along the way, you can add squats, lunges, and knee lifts, then add some arm movements to get a full body warm-up.

Introducing the dynamic warm-up

This involves spending a few minutes on an overall body warm-up, then taking some time to focus on exercises specific to your sport or activity. Use activities and movement patterns that are similar to those in your chosen workout and do them at a slower pace and with less intensity at first.

Gradually increase speed and intensity across your warm-up but remember to take it easy. Your warm-up should leave you slightly sweaty and ready to go – not slumped over and completely worn out.

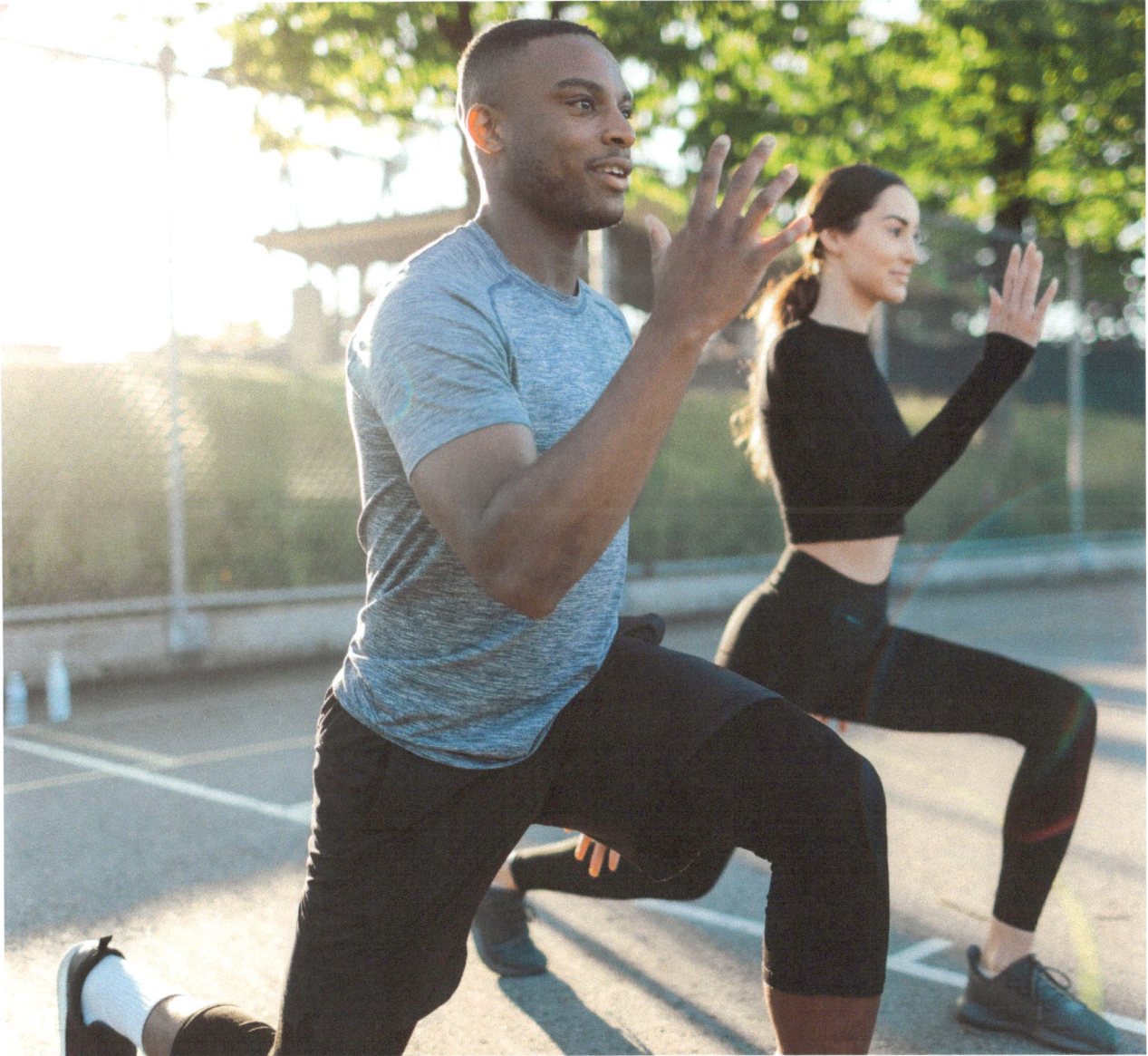

NOTES

Believe. Train. Nourish. Achieve.

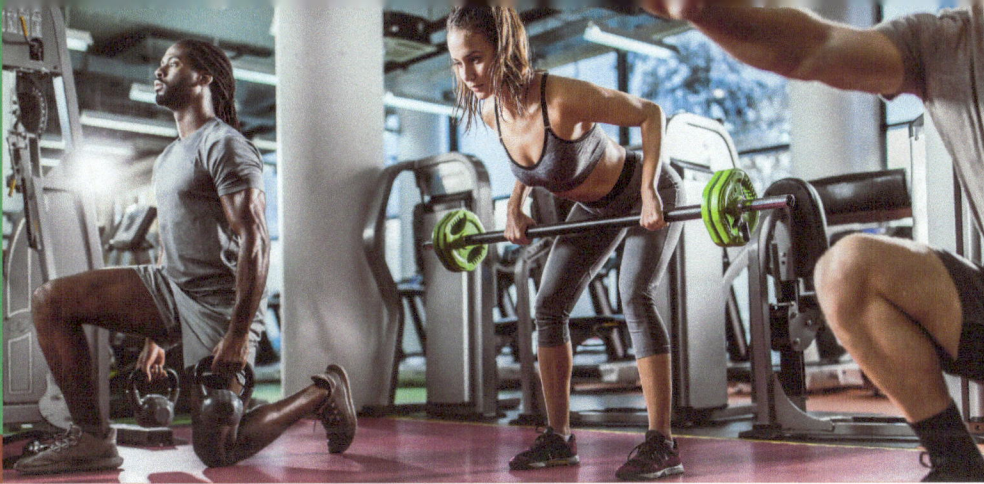

Training

I am building a fire, and every day I train, I add more fuel.

Mia Hamm

When you've got a clear goal, and you're committed to putting in the hours of training required, you want to make sure that you're getting the most out of your training.

Here are some practical steps to maximise the benefits of your training

1. Incorporate a healthy balance of cardio and strength training

It's tempting to fill all your training sessions with the type of exercise you love. Runners, for example, are notorious for focusing solely on running. If left to their own devices, many of them will completely ignore strength training, yoga or Pilates. Some gym fanatics are just as bad, spending all their time pumping iron and never setting foot on a treadmill.

Scientists have found that focusing solely on either cardio or strength, actually sabotages your training. You'll get far greater benefit from a program that includes a variety of exercise types.

If you are new to training or returning after a long absence, look for a full-body workout that includes a balance of cardio and strength training. This will yield optimal results for all fitness goals.

When you're starting out with strength training, remember to start slow.

Where possible, beginners should use the weight machines in the gym to learn the correct form for each exercise. Only move on to free weights once you've gained strength and confidence.

That said, training with free weights, such as dumbbells, kettlebells, and barbells, is a good ultimate goal, as it has been shown to generate greater hormonal responses than training on gym equipment. This is because free weight training, without anything to guide or support your movement, taps into a larger range of muscles.

Only use weights that you can comfortably do 12 to 15 reps with. Ideally, you should aim to complete 3 sets of 12 reps of each type of exercise. Later, you can increase this to 3 sets of 15 reps.

As a rule of thumb, if, when pushing those last few reps, you feel you could keep going, you're probably ready to try the same exercise with a slightly heavier weight next time. Alternatively, you could stay at the same weight and do more reps per set, depending on your goals – ask a fitness professional to find out which option is right for you.

As you progress with strength training, you'll be able to do separate upper- and lower-body training sessions on alternating days.

And, once you are comfortably able to manage it, you could move on to a full split approach in which you train specific muscle groups each day. Depending on your goals, this could involve doing up to 20 reps per set.

2. Pump up the jams

Listening to your favourite playlist is a great way to put yourself in the mood for a workout. Just make sure that the music doesn't interfere with your mindfulness while exercising. You should still be able to be fully present and focus on your workout with the music playing in the background.

Also, try listening to some relaxing tunes while you cool down. Studies indicate that listening to music boosts the body's serotonin and dopamine levels, and these hormones promote faster recovery. Listening to music also helps to get blood pressure and heart rate back to normal, which speeds up recovery.

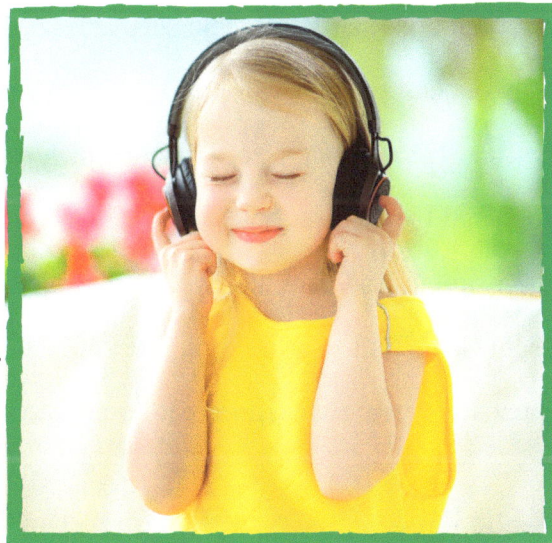

3. Embrace interval training

Interval training consists of short bursts of high-intensity exercises followed by periods of lower-intensity exercise. For example, 20 seconds of jogging as fast as you can on the spot, followed by 30 seconds of marching on the spot or 30 seconds of burpees followed by 30 reps of tricep dips.

The intense bursts of exercise performed at maximum effort during interval training sessions get your heart rate up and keep it up throughout your workout. This approach rapidly improves cardiovascular fitness, triggers fat loss, and sculpts the body faster than other workouts.

Your body continues to burn calories for hours after you've completed an interval training session as it works through a range of functions to recover from the intense exercise.

As a result, interval training has been scientifically proven to burn more calories per minute than other workout types – yes, even running.

Popular versions of interval training include HIIT (high-intensity interval training) and Tabata. Beginner HIIT programs typically consist of whole-body exercise sequences that alternate between body parts to enable adequate rest and recovery. More advanced HIIT sessions might focus only on legs and glutes one day, and on arms, abs, and core the next.

Tabata is a type of HIIT in which each set consists of 20 seconds of flat-out intensity, followed by a 10-second rest period. A round of Tabata usually consists of just four exercises, and the workout isn't over until you've completed eight sets of each exercise. At first glance, Tabata may seem easy, but it *is* challenging. If you're new to exercise, older, or have been injured, consider low-intensity steady-state (LISS) cardio instead.

4. Mix things up with low-intensity steady-state cardio (LISS)

These sessions are the opposite of HIIT training sessions. While hard and fast HIIT training is great for burning fat and building stamina, LISS sessions provide a slow and steady approach to getting fitter and leaner. In HIIT, you're going hard in short bursts, whereas with LISS you're exercising at a steady, sustained pace over a longer period of time.

LISS sessions are great for burning calories and improving cardiovascular health. The steady pace means your heart rate will be elevated to 50% to 65% of your maximum heart rate (MHR).

Your MHR is the upper limit of what your cardiovascular system can tolerate, and it is calculated using the following formula.

220 – your age = your MHR in beats per minute (bpm)

If you multiply your MHR by 0.5 and 0.65, you'll get the upper and lower limits of your heart rate during LISS, respectively. If possible, use a smartwatch or heart rate monitor to track your heart rate while you exercise and try to keep it in this range by slowing down or resting if it gets beyond the upper limit and pushing a little more if it drops below your lower limit. This will ensure that your heart rate and effort levels remain within a safe and sustainable range throughout your workout.

LISS sessions should last for 30 to 60 minutes, depending on how fit you are. If you are a beginner, it's best to start with 30 to 40 minutes and gradually increase to 60 minutes as you get fitter.

LISS cardio jumpstarts a number of positive reactions in the body including maximising the amount of oxygen in the blood and raising the heart rate to promote healthy blood flow to the heart and muscles.

The American Council on Exercise has established that regular sustained low-intensity exercise improves cardiorespiratory fitness, extends aerobic capacity, reduces the risk of major chronic illnesses, supports bodily functions, and promotes health.

LISS is also great for weight loss as it provides the oxygen required to convert fat into energy. The extended exercise time of LISS helps the body become more efficient at using body fat rather than muscle glycogen stores for energy and keeps it burning fat for longer.

LISS has been shown to be more effective than HIIT at improving weight distribution in overweight adults. And, it reduces the build-up of visceral fat that collects around the organs and causes chronic disease.

This slow-and-steady approach to training is ideal for beginners, older adults, and those with persistent injuries, allowing them to form regular exercise habits without pushing their bodies beyond their limits.

Similarly, LISS results in fewer injuries as it is low impact and therefore kinder to the joints and muscles. In fact, it is so gentle that you can do it every day without the risk of sore muscles.

LISS also improves mood by stimulating the release of feel-good neurotransmitters, such as dopamine and serotonin.

Examples of LISS workouts include:

- Walking at a comfortable pace for 30 to 60 minutes.
- Jogging slowly for 30 to 45 minutes.
- Cycling on flat terrain or using a stationary bike at a gentle speed for 30 to 60 minutes.
- Swimming breaststroke for 30 minutes.
- Using a rowing machine at a consistent rate and intensity for 30 minutes or more.

5. Start with carbs, end with protein

We'll be going into nutrition in more detail in the next section of this book, but for now, we'll share a couple of quick and easy tips that will help you power through your workouts. For starters, topping up your carbohydrate levels by eating a light snack, such as a bowl of oatmeal or an energy bar, just before a workout can help you fuel your body for success, particularly during high-intensity workouts. With the proper fuel, your body will be able to perform better, and you'll burn more calories and build more muscle.

As soon as you can after a high-intensity or long-duration workout, finish off your training session with a protein-rich snack. This will speed up recovery and sustain muscle growth. Low-fat chocolate milk is a popular post-workout snack because it contains a good balance (4:1) of carbs to protein. Carbs help restore your energy levels, and proteins stimulate muscle repair.

Quick tip Eating a protein-rich snack, especially one rich in casein such as Greek yoghurt or cottage cheese, just before bed also helps build your muscles back up after an intense workout. In fact, these slow-digesting casein-rich snacks keep amino acid and muscle protein synthesis rates high throughout the night.

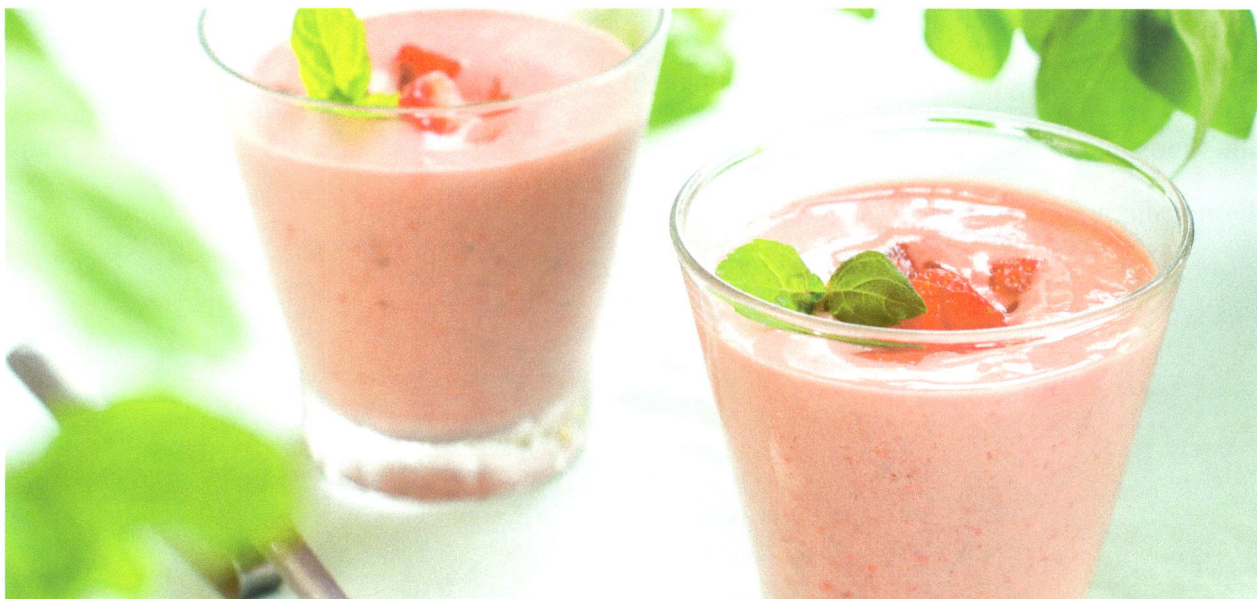

6. Stay hydrated

No health and fitness tip has ever been touted more often than this simple call to drink more water. And yet, it remains one of the tips most often disregarded. Aside from reducing the effectiveness of your workout, not paying attention to hydration can make your workout feel harder, diminish your performance, and hamper your body's ability to recover.

Depending on how heavily you tend to sweat when you're working out, you could be losing between 2% and 10% of your body weight in fluids. Worse still, many gym-goers (and others) are dehydrated before they even start their workouts. This can have devastating effects on your health.

Experts recommend that as a general rule, your daily water requirements can be calculated using the equation:

$$\text{Water (litres)} = \text{Body weight (kg)} \times 0.033$$

Stay safe by weighing yourself before and after your training session. If you've been hydrating properly, you should not have lost more than 2% of your body weight during the session. If you've lost more than this, top up your water levels as soon as possible, and remember to drink more during your next training session.

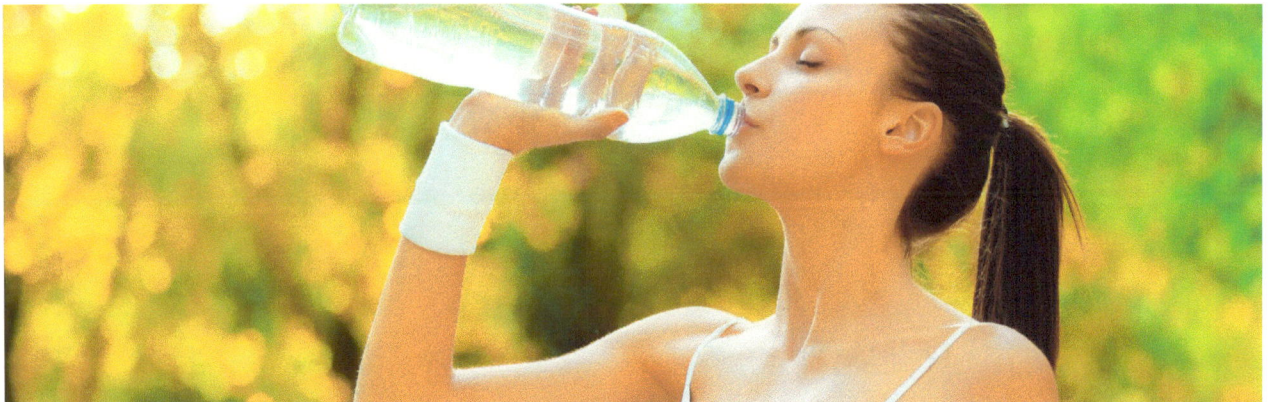

7. Rest and recovery are just as important as working out

Don't skip your rest days. They are just as important as your workout days. Your muscles don't get stronger and fitter during your workouts – they do this after workouts, during the recovery phase. Taking a rest day once a week gives your muscles time to recover, so you can come back stronger for your next workout.

We'll be taking a closer look at rest and sleep in the next chapter, but we want to mention here how important it is to get seven to nine hours of good quality sleep every night.

The hormone changes that happen while you sleep promote recovery. Without a good night's rest, you're likely to experience symptoms of over-training, and your fitness may plateau. A lack of proper sleep has also been shown to reduce your ability to perform exercises with proper form, which affects the number of calories you burn during a workout.

8. Make time for a massage

Massage, either by a professional sports physio or at home using a foam roller or massage ball, plays an important role in assisting your body to recover and grow stronger. It activates the genes in your muscle cells, decreasing inflammation and increasing the number of mitochondria. *Mito what?* Mitochondria are microscopic structures in your cells that help to power your muscles during exercise and recovery. So, the more mitochondria, the better for your cells.

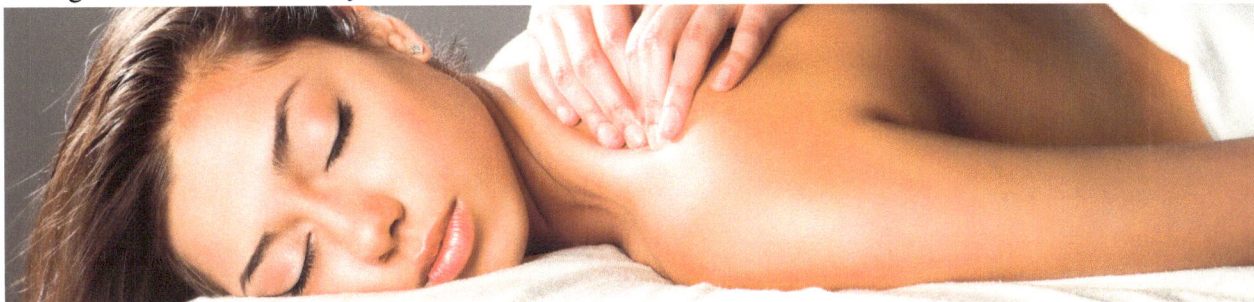

NOTES

Believe. Train. Nourish. Achieve.

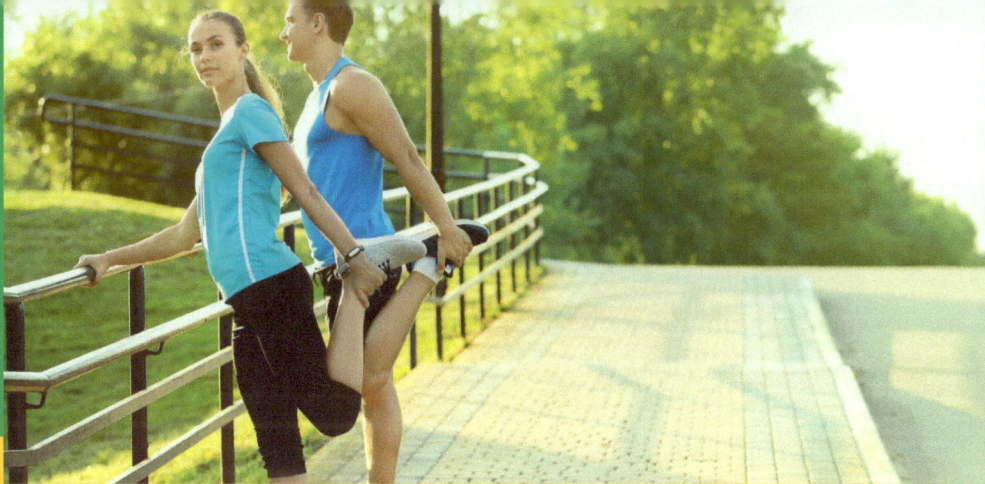

Cooling down

The importance of the warm-up and the cool-down cannot be stressed enough.

Jamie Redknapp

Why take the time to cool down?

A proper cool-down session has both psychological and physiological benefits. It helps to regulate blood flow, gradually lowers your heart rate and blood pressure, and allows your body to slowly recover and return to its pre-exercise state.

So, instead of rushing off to get on with your day, honour your body and the work you've done during your training session by spending some time cooling down.

How to cool down properly

Cooling down is best done directly after your workout session. It only takes 5 to 10 minutes, but the benefits are enormous. Plus, it's really easy. Simply repeat the exercises you did in your warm-up session. Or do a slower, less intense form of the exercise you did during your training session. For example, to cool down after swimming training, swim a few laps at a leisurely pace for 5 to 10 minutes.

Stretching

Stretching improves the flexibility and mobility of your joints and can help improve performance by allowing your joints to move through their full range of motion.

Research indicates that stretching is best kept for *after* your warm-up or just before your cool-down sessions when muscles and tendons are warm and supple. Vigorously stretching cold muscles and ligaments can lead to injury. Even with warm muscles, you should only stretch to the point where it is comfortable. Listen to your body and don't try to push past pain or force a stretch.

A good way to safely stretch and improve your strength and mobility would be to get advice from you gym or personal trainer or to add Pilates or yoga classes to your fitness program.

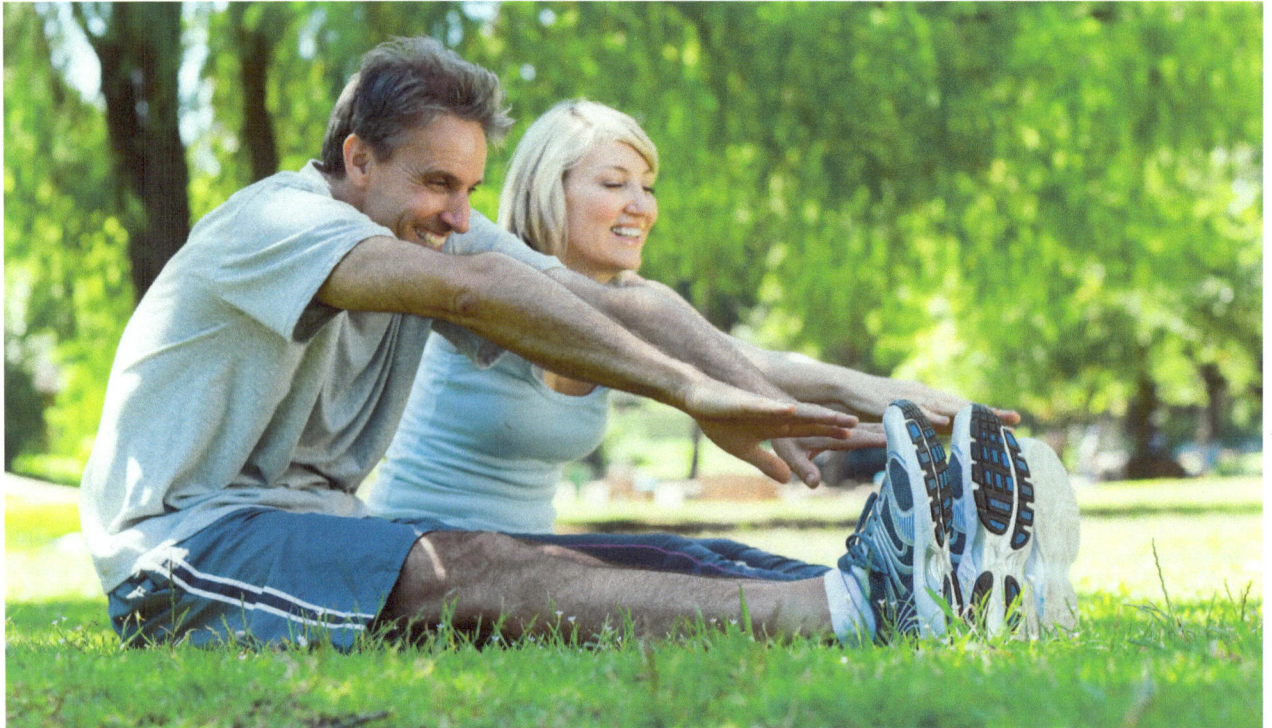

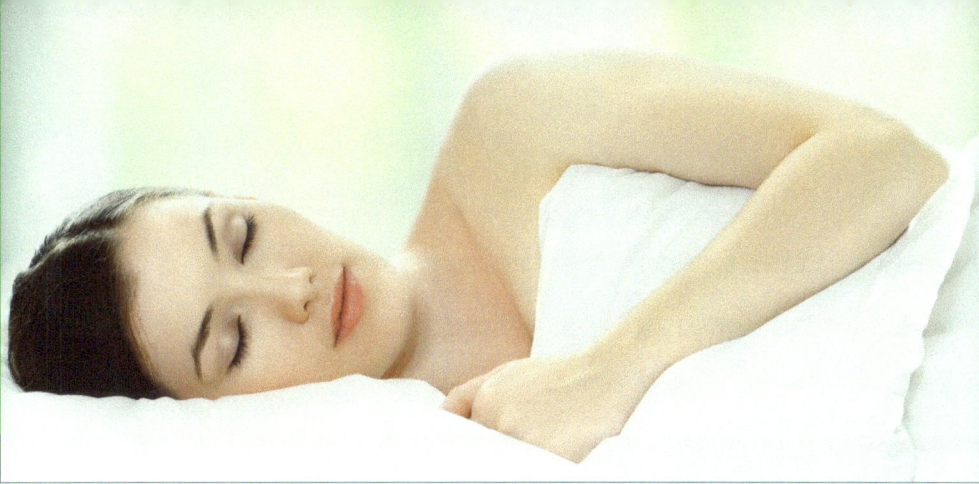

Sleep and rest

You can make excuses for why you don't or can't sleep – or you can sleep and ensure
that all your time, effort, and energy is leading to the day you have dreamed about.
John Underwood

It's common knowledge that human beings perform better after they've had a good night's sleep and, in recent years, this age-old fact of life has been scientifically proven many times over.

Despite all the evidence pointing to the importance of sleep, we frequently downplay the role of sleep in our lives. Technology, eating habits, unprecedented stress levels, and the pressure to squeeze as many activities as possible into 24 hours all cause us to sacrifice sleep, both in terms of duration and quality.

How sleep happens

Before the 1950s, people thought the brain and body were dormant during sleep, but now we know that sleep is much more than just a passive period during your day. While you sleep, your brain is busy with a number of necessary life-sustaining activities, all of which affect the quality of your waking life.

The sleep cycle

There are two different types of sleep that your brain cycles through repeatedly while you are asleep. These are known as REM (rapid eye movement) and non-REM sleep.

Non-REM sleep

The sleep cycle begins with non-REM sleep, which is composed of four stages:

Stage 1: Between being awake and falling asleep.

Stage 2: Light sleep. Your heart rate and breathing are regulated, and your body temperature drops.

Stage 3 and 4: Deep sleep stages that lead into REM sleep.

Each sleep cycle typically lasts 90 to 120 minutes, and the cycle usually repeats four or five times during the night. With each cycle, you spend less time in non-REM Stages 3 and 4, and more time in REM sleep.

Until recently, REM sleep was thought to be the most important part of the sleep cycle. But, current studies indicate that non-REM sleep is the more restful and restorative part of sleep and is more important for learning and memory.

REM sleep

During the REM part of the sleep cycle, your eyeballs move rapidly beneath your eyelids. Brain waves in this cycle are similar to those measured when awake, breathing increases, and your body becomes temporarily paralysed while you dream.

What controls your urge to sleep?

Two main processes regulate sleep: circadian rhythms and sleep drive.

Circadian rhythms are controlled by a dedicated area in your brain that responds to lower light levels by releasing the sleep hormone melatonin.

Sleep drive works very much the same way as your hunger drive does. Your desire for sleep builds throughout the day, and, when your craving for sleep reaches a certain point, the need to sleep can no longer be ignored.

Unlike hunger, where you are still more or less in control, your sleep drive maxes out at a point where you are no longer able to control the urge to sleep. Your body takes over and forces you to drift off. If you've ever felt yourself dozing in the classroom or at work, you'll know how impossible it is to stay awake at this point.

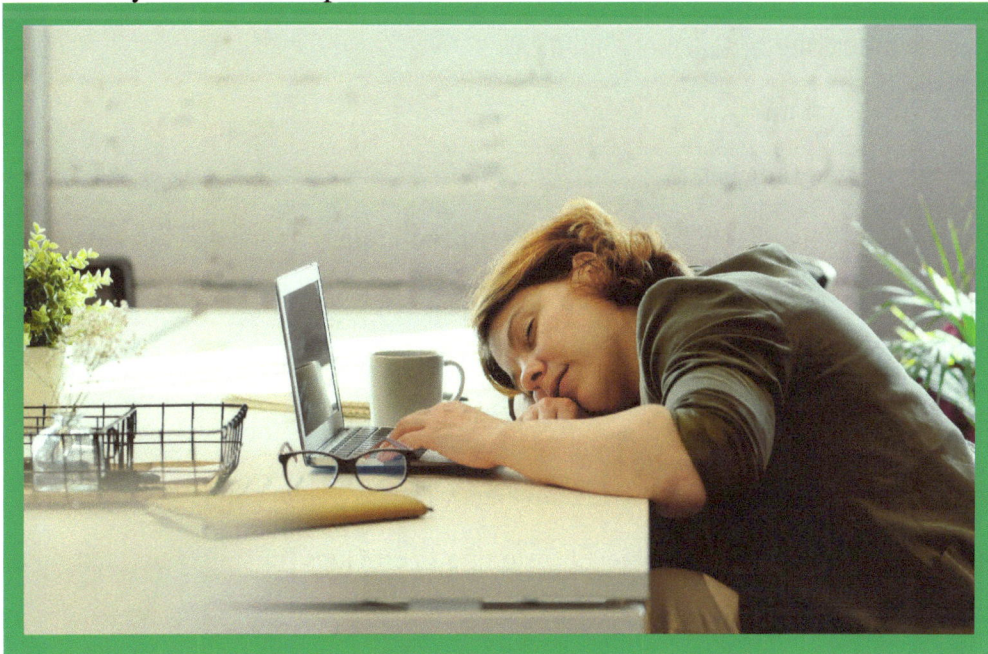

Why is sleep so important?

Studies indicate that quality sleep has profound effects on performance, training outcomes, and recovery times.

A lack of proper sleep has multiple negative effects including:

1. Reduced performance.

2. Reduced cardiovascular fitness.

3. Lower endurance.

4. Reduced muscle formation.

5. Lower tolerance for high-intensity workouts.

6. Reduced skill acquisition.

7. Reduced reaction times.

8. Slower decision-making and memory abilities.

9. Slower recovery from injury.

10. Increased risk of type II diabetes.

    a. Just one night of missed sleep can create a pre-diabetic state – even in a healthy person.

11. Increased weight gain.

    a. Getting less than seven hours of sleep per night has been shown to increase the levels of ghrelin – the hormone that makes you feel hungry – and lower the levels of leptin – the hormone that makes you feel full. This imbalance causes you to feel hungrier and overeat.

    b. Lack of sleep leads to low energy levels resulting in cravings for sugary and fatty foods.

12. Increased incidence of migraines.

13. Increased fatigue, lethargy, and lack of motivation to work out or do any of the activities you usually enjoy.

14. Increased risk of depression.

15. Increased levels of inflammation that increase your risk of developing chronic medical conditions, such as heart disease and Alzheimer's disease.

16. Increased risk of death or injury.

On the other hand, getting plenty of good quality sleep has been shown to improve your mental and physical performance, boost your immune system, and enhance your reaction times, muscular power and endurance, and fine motor and problem-solving skills. Along with exercise and nutrition, taking care of your sleep health by prioritising sleep is essential.

Just remember, sleep is training too!

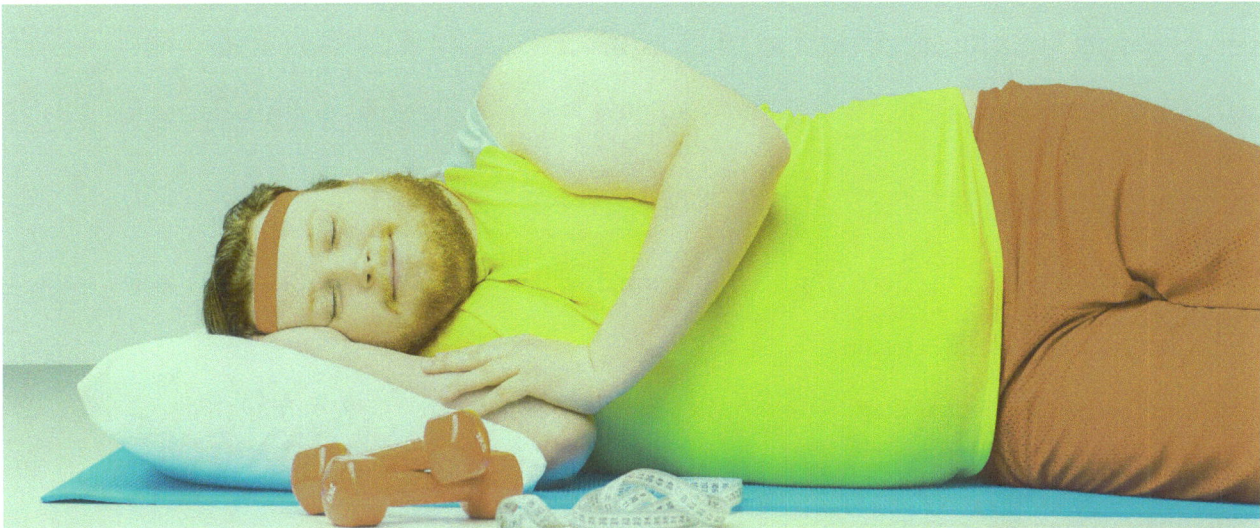

How to improve your sleep hygiene and get a good night's rest

1. Create the right environment for sleep

Good sleep hygiene is essential to improve the quality, duration, and regularity of your sleep. **It all starts with creating the optimum environment that will make it easy to get quality sleep:**

- Your bedroom should be a cool, dark, quiet, technology-free zone.
- Keep your bedroom clear of all other stimuli, which means absolutely no working or studying in bed and no visual stimuli, such as social media, videos or TV in bed.
- Your bed should be fitted out for sleep with a quality mattress, and enough sheets, pillows, and blankets to keep your body at a comfortable temperature – neither too hot nor too cold.

2. Set aside enough time for proper sleep

Sleep duration is very important. Try to get between seven and nine hours of uninterrupted sleep per night. This should increase to 10 hours of sleep per night for top athletes. Give yourself more hours of sleep per night at times when your days are particularly physically demanding.

3. Create and maintain a sleep routine

Maintain your circadian rhythms by developing a consistent sleep routine. This means going to bed and waking up at the same times every day.

Ensure you get good quality undisturbed sleep by taking care of everything that requires your attention and getting as much as possible ready for the following day, before going to bed.

For example, get your workout gear ready, select your work clothes, and pack your lunch box for the next day.

Avoid sugar and caffeine late in the day. Make sure that you've had enough (but not too much) to eat, and that you're properly hydrated before heading off to bed.

4. Create and stick to a 30-minute pre-sleep wind-down

Your sleep routine should include approximately 30 minutes of wind-down time. Switch off and avoid using technology, such as TV, phones, laptops, computers, and any devices that emit stimulating blue light during your wind-down time, as this light interferes with your ability to fall asleep. Take care of your physical needs, such as cleaning your teeth and going to the toilet, during your wind-down time.

5. Settle down and relax

Once you're in bed and ready to sleep, avoid looking at bright lights, such as your bedside clock or phone. Use a sleep mask to block out any residual light. Close your eyes, focus on your breathing, and use relaxation techniques or listen to guided sleep meditations to help you settle down.

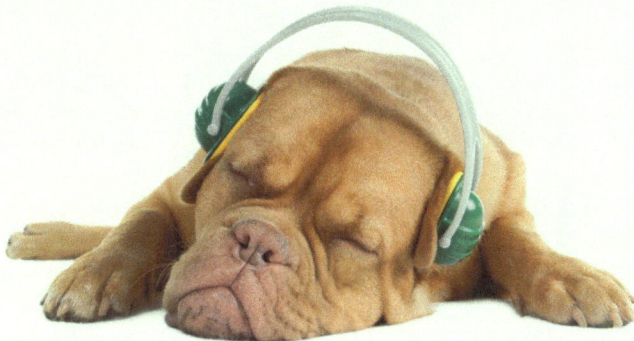

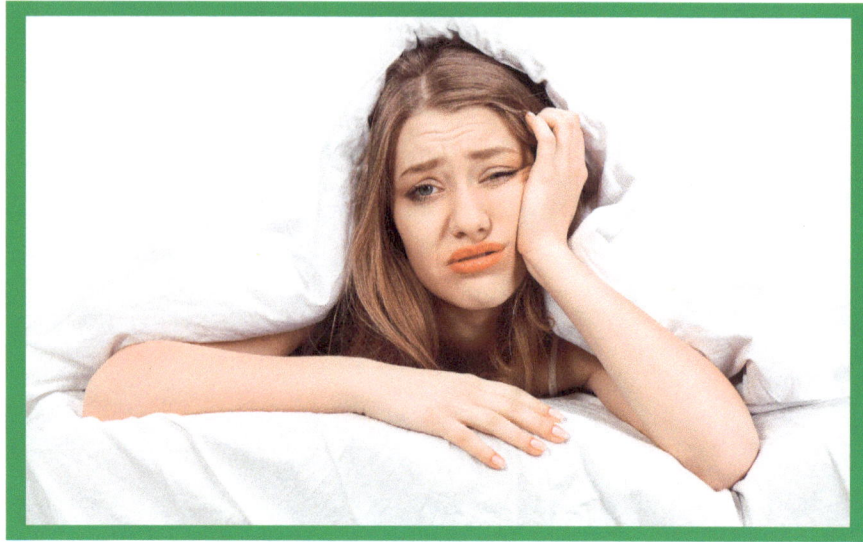

What to do if you can't fall asleep

If you are struggling to sleep, try not to panic or obsess over it. The more you chase sleep, the further it runs from you.

Instead, acknowledge and accept that you don't feel like sleeping, and tell yourself it's okay not to sleep; it's fine to just rest, relax, and lie still for a while. There's no need to do anything right now. Keep your eyes closed, focus on your breath, and just let go. Sleep will come when you least expect it.

If you're still awake after 20 to 30 minutes, get up and do something calming or monotonous while avoiding bright lights, smartphones, TV, and computers. For example, you could try listening to some soothing music or an audiobook that's not too cerebral, doing a guided meditation or reading a printed book in low light. You could even try knitting or crocheting – any thing you can do on autopilot. Now's not the time to take up a new hobby or learn a new skill.

Sleep debt – how can you pay it back?

If you're feeling fuzzy and fatigued due to lack of sleep, here are a couple of ways that you can recoup lost sleep.

Napping

A 30-minute post-lunch nap is recommended for paying back sleep debt and improving your short-term performance – especially when you have afternoon or evening training sessions or matches. Just watch out: daytime napping for more than 30 minutes can rob you of your ability to sleep in the evening by throwing your circadian rhythms out of whack.

Increasing sleep duration

We are all well acquainted with the rejuvenating effects of the occasional sleep-in. Unfortunately, one-off increases in sleep have only limited benefits as far as improving performance and reducing sleep debt. One to two hours more sleep every night for a couple of weeks is needed before any real benefits become evident.

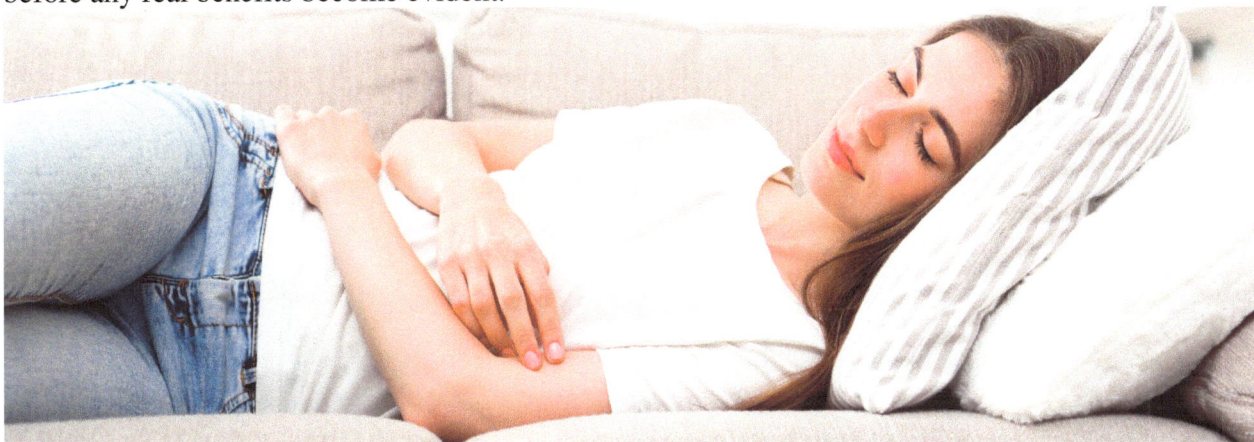

NOTES

Believe. Train. Nourish. Achieve.

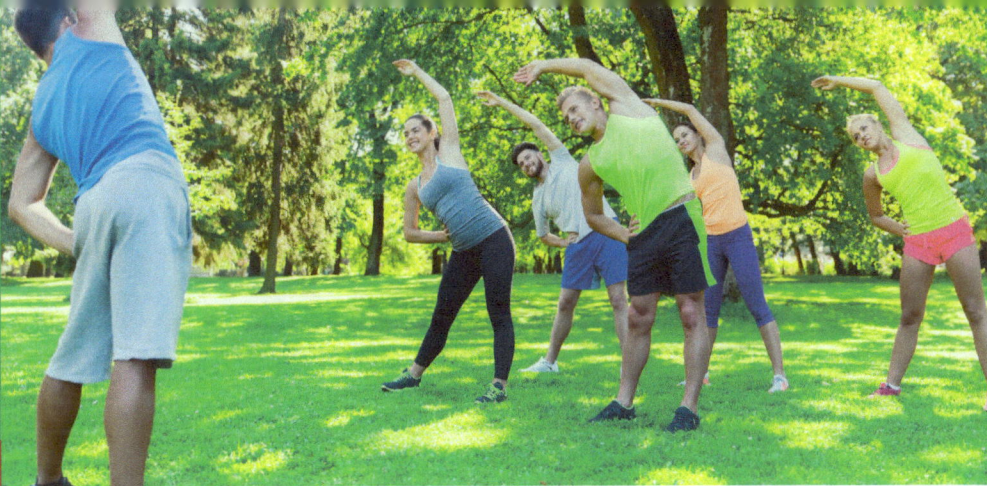

Getting back to training

If you're returning to fitness training after a long absence, whether due to physical restrictions, such as quarantine or isolation, or recovery from illness, a medical condition, childbirth, surgery or injury, it goes without saying that you need to take a different approach to your training than an already fit person would. Here are a few points to consider when starting back up again.

Don't rely on past performance

Don't expect to hop back in where you left off when returning to exercise after a long break. Eighteen months ago, you may have jumped out of bed each morning and gone for a 10 km run but busting out 10 km after such a long break would hurt – a lot.

Waiting for your body to catch up to its previous performance levels can be hard, especially if you have been a highly active person and have been sedentary for a long time due to ill health or injury. Feelings of anger and frustration often bubble up when a fit and active identity is in conflict with the body's current inability to function as it once did. This might tempt you to "push through the pain" and keep going. But, pushing yourself too hard too soon, could leave you feeling demotivated and disappointed by your performance. It could even lead to further injury. And you know what that means? *More* recovery time and longer periods of inactivity before you can start up again. Instead, be patient with your body, acknowledge that it has been through a lot, and gently coax yourself back into a regular training program.

Honest self-evaluation and acceptance of your body in its current state will allow you to set realistic and achievable fitness goals that suit your present abilities. You'll be exercising safely and growing fitter and stronger, and you'll be more motivated to keep going.

Start slow and build up

When returning to exercise, you'll need to start slow and build back up again. Speak to your doctor, physiotherapist, coach or trainer to determine which exercises will have the greatest impact on your recovery and work within their recommendations. Avoid the temptation to add reps, sets or exercises without consulting a fitness professional first. This will ensure that you're staying safe and helping your body get stronger.

Mix things up a little

When you're getting back into things, it helps to vary the intensity, frequency, and type of exercise you are doing. Not only does this reduce boredom and make it easier to stay motivated, but it also helps your body to recover quicker.

Our bodies respond better to a variety of different moves than they do to the same moves being repeated over and over. That's why cross-training, which involves a balance of cardio, strength, and stretching exercises, is so important for building strength and endurance and reducing the risk of injury.

Strength exercises are especially important as weak muscles can lead to joint pain when you're exercising. The older you are, the more important it becomes to include strength training in your program.

Don't forget the proven benefits of LISS discussed in the Training chapter. This type of low-intensity steady-state exercise is ideal to boost your fitness levels without placing too much stress on the body when you're getting back into exercise.

Choose the types of training that you enjoy

To keep yourself motivated, even when the going gets tough, try to choose exercises and activities that you enjoy. If you love cardio, but hate jogging, make sure your training program includes alternative cardio exercises, such as aerobics, swimming or cycling. Discuss your preferences with your coach, trainer, physiotherapist or doctor to ensure your options are safe and stay within your recovery program.

Consistency and perseverance are key

It can be disheartening when you first get back into fitness training to see little or no real improvement. Don't give up or give in to excuses. It's time for perseverance. With consistent, sustained effort you'll start to see results. In the meantime, you just have to get out there and do the work. The easiest way to ensure perseverance and consistency is to make your new training program part of your daily routine. Do it every day, regardless of what you see on the scale or how motivated you feel.

If you keep anything up day after day for long enough, it will become a habit – just like brushing your teeth. Try thinking of your training routine in the same way as your other daily habits, i.e., as something you simply do each day, no matter what (at least in the beginning stages).

The day will come when, finally, your perseverance has paid off, and you're starting to see results. The needle moves on the scale, your performance improves or you find that you're actually enjoying your workouts. Suddenly, training changes from being something you just do, to something you love to do.

Focus on progress, not perfection.

Another important mindset shift for those returning to exercise after a long absence is to focus on progress, not perfection. For example, if you set out to complete a parkrun, and end up running only two-thirds of the way, instead of running the whole way as planned, don't beat yourself up about it. Celebrate your progress. Congratulate yourself on running two-thirds of the way when a few weeks ago you weren't even able to run one-third of the way.

Don't go throwing in the towel just because you had a bad workout or even a bad week of workouts. Keep going and persevere. If you've had a string of bad workouts in a row – at least you've been working out.

The important thing to remember is you're playing the long game. Your progress may be slow, but it's steady, and it's getting you closer to your goal each day. As that classic 80s poster said, 'Hang in there!' Things will improve.

Rest and recovery

Regardless of the workout program you're following, rest days are crucial when returning to fitness. They give your body time to heal and your muscles a chance to grow stronger and get ready for your next workout.

If you have accidentally overdone it, and you're feeling a little sore after your workout, it's even more important for you to take time off to rest and recover.

Follow the RICE procedure, which stands for Rest, Ice, Compression, Elevation, to treat any injuries and hold off on the exercise until the symptoms have cleared up.

If the injury is severe, involves joint swelling, and cannot bear weight, or if a mild injury persists for a week or more, it's time to see a healthcare professional.

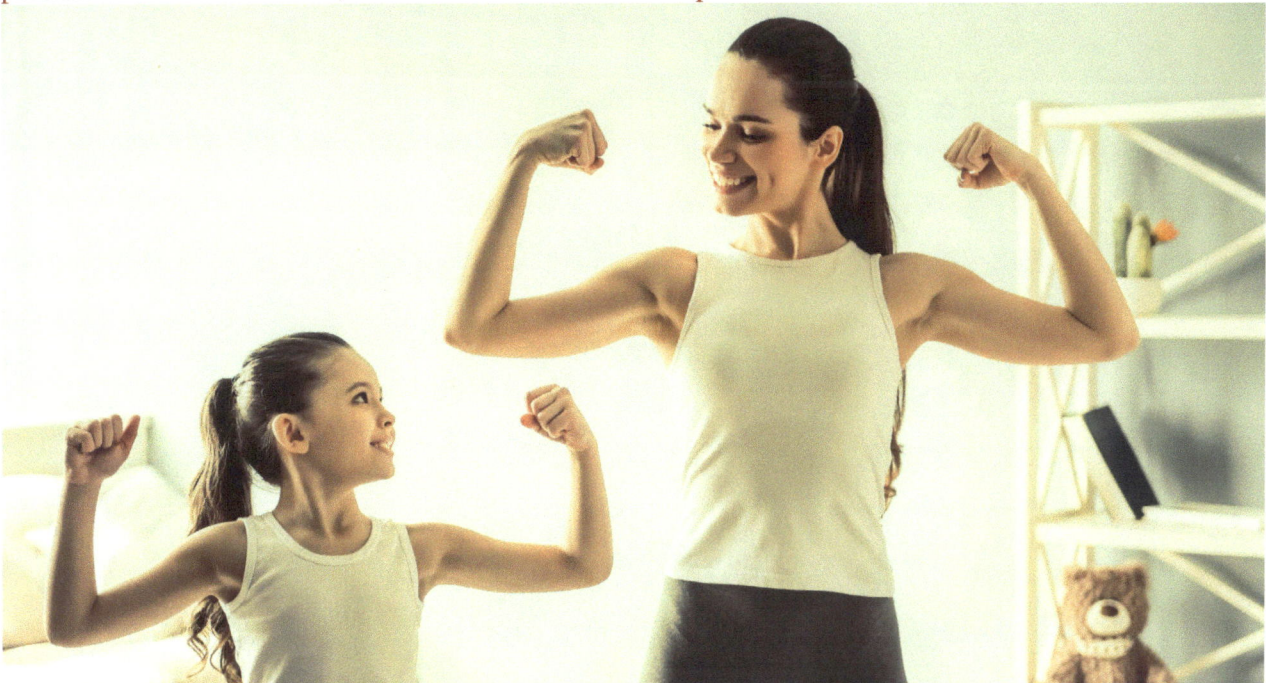

NOTES

Believe. Train. Nourish. Achieve.

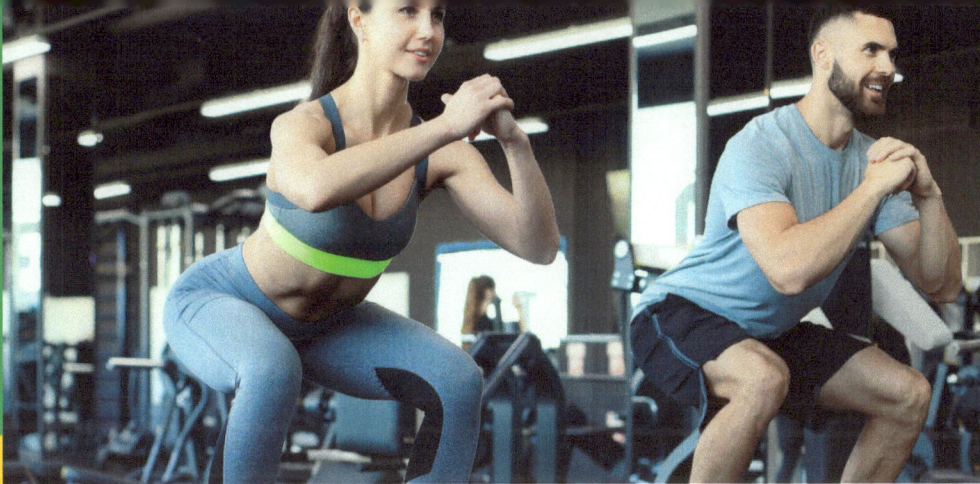

Bonus
Training programs

The following training programs have been designed by fitness professionals, Jo and Johnny Black. They are general in nature and are to be used as a guide only.

Do not attempt these or any new fitness program without first consulting your healthcare professional to determine its suitability for you.

We also strongly recommend consulting a fitness professional prior to starting any of these training programs to ensure that they are suitable for your particular goals, needs, and fitness levels.

If you are unfamiliar with any of the exercises mentioned below, please ask your fitness trainer for advice on how to do them safely and effectively.

Warm up and cool down

We've included examples of warm-up and cool-down routines that you could do before and after your workouts, respectively.

WARM UP

EXERCISE	TIME
Light cardio such as marching/jogging on the spot or stationary bike (in a low gear)	5 to 10 minutes
• Arm reaches • Side reaches • Hip rotations • Knee lifts • Lateral lunges • Lateral lunges with ankle touches • Squats • Squat and reach up • Grapevines	20 to 30 seconds each

Believe. Train. Nourish. Achieve.

COOL DOWN & STRETCHES

EXERCISE	TIME
Light cardio such as marching/jogging on the spot or stationary bike (in a low gear)	5 to 10 minutes
• Standing quad stretch (each leg) • Lunging calf stretch (each leg) • Seated single leg hamstring stretch (each leg) • Core abdominal stretch • Child's pose • Downward dog stretch • Double knee-to-chest stretch • Single knee-to-chest stretch (each side) • Bent knee cross-body stretch (each side) • Folded-4 stretch or seated pigeon stretch (each side) • Piriformis stretch (each side) • Triceps stretch (each arm) • Shoulder stretch (each arm) • Spinal twist (each side)	Hold each stretch for 20 to 30 seconds
Foam rolling and trigger point release	5 to 10 minutes

Training program 1

Scalable three-day home circuit program

Body weight three-day circuit

This program can be done at home, requires no equipment, and can be scaled to suit your fitness level, whether beginner, intermediate or advanced.

Beginner

- Start with the minimum repetitions and work your way up to the maximum repetitions.
- Only do what you feel comfortable with each time and work up until you are able to complete one round of the workout comfortably.
- Make sure you have a rest day between workouts and take two rest days after Day 3, before starting with Day 1 again. For example, do Workout 1 on Monday, Rest Tuesday, Workout 2 on Wednesday, Rest Thursday, Workout 3 on Friday, Rest over the weekend, and start again on Monday with Workout 1.

Intermediate

- Start with the minimum repetitions and work your way up to the maximum repetitions.
- Only do what you feel comfortable with each time and work up until you are able to complete two rounds of the workout comfortably.

Intermediate (cont.)

- Make sure you have a rest day between workouts and take two rest days after Day 3, before starting with Day 1 again. For example, do Workout 1 on Monday, Rest Tuesday, Workout 2 on Wednesday, Rest Thursday, Workout 3 on Friday, Rest over the weekend, and start again on Monday with Workout 1.

Advanced

- Start with the minimum repetitions and work your way up to the maximum repetitions.
- Only do what you feel comfortable with each time and work up until you are able to complete three rounds of the workout comfortably.
- Make sure you have a rest day between workouts and take two rest days after Day 3, before starting with Day 1 again. For example, do Workout 1 on Monday, Rest Tuesday, Workout 2 on Wednesday, Rest Thursday, Workout 3 on Friday, Rest over the weekend, and start again on Monday with Workout 1.

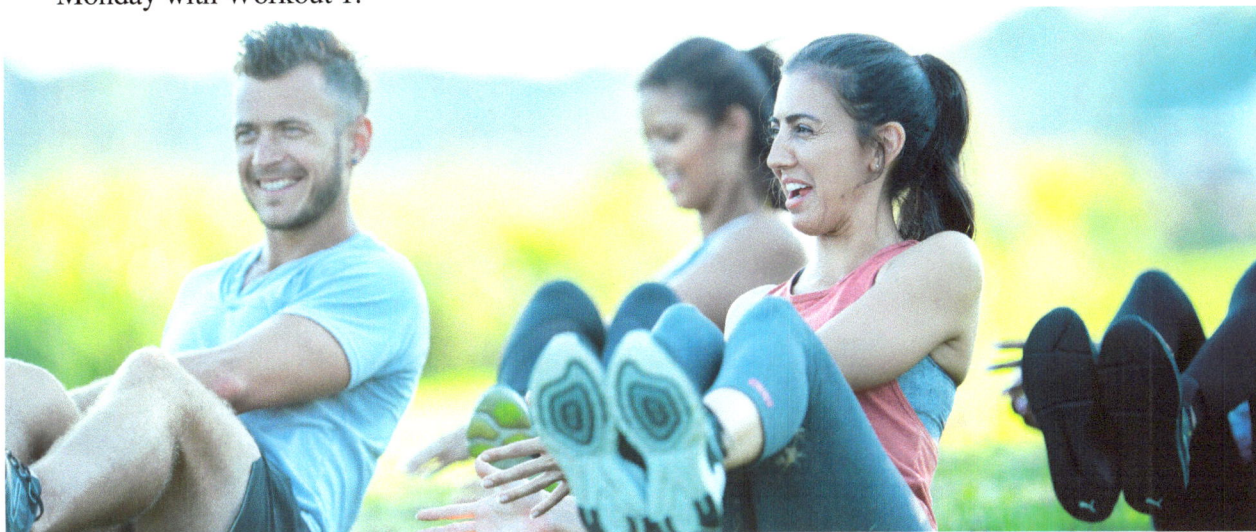

Scalable three-day home circuit program

	EXERCISES	REPETITIONS/ DURATION	BREAKS BETWEEN EXERCISES
WORKOUT 1	Jump squats	6–8	40 seconds
	Burpees	6–8	40 seconds
	Lateral squats	10 per side	40 seconds
	Stationary lunges	10 per side	30 seconds
	Push-ups (on toes/knees)	12	30 seconds
	Bench (tricep) dips	12	30 seconds
	Mountain climbers	20 seconds	30 seconds
	Crunches	20 seconds	30 seconds
	Reverse crunches	20 seconds	30 seconds
	Plank	30–60 seconds	30 seconds

Training program 1

Scalable three-day home circuit program

	EXERCISES	REPETITIONS/ DURATION	BREAKS BETWEEN EXERCISES
WORKOUT 2	Jumping jacks	15 seconds	30 seconds
	High knees	15 seconds	30 seconds
	Burpees	6–8	30 seconds
	Step-up (Use a step, chair or bench)	8–10	30 seconds
	Squats	15	30 seconds
	Push-ups (on toes/knees)	15	30 seconds
	Reverse crunches	20 seconds	20 seconds
	Side plank	20 seconds	20 seconds
	Side plank hip raises	20 seconds	20 seconds

Training program 1

Scalable three-day home circuit program

	EXERCISES	REPETITIONS/ DURATION	BREAKS BETWEEN EXERCISES
WORKOUT 3	Run/jog on the spot	15 seconds	30 seconds
	Mountain climbers	15 seconds	30 seconds
	Burpees	6–8	30 seconds
	Lateral lunges	8–10	30 seconds
	Floor IYT raises	6–8	30 seconds
	Push-ups (on toes/knees)	15	30 seconds
	Table-top crunches	30 seconds	15 seconds
	Plank	30–60 seconds	20 seconds
	Side plank hip raises	20 seconds	20 seconds
	Leg raises	30 seconds	30 seconds

Training program 2

Intermediate three-day gym circuit program

- Start with the minimum repetitions and work your way up to the maximum repetitions.

- Only do what you feel comfortable with each time and work up until you are able to complete two rounds of the workout comfortably.

- Make sure you have a rest day between workouts and two rest days after Day 3.

	EXERCISES	SETS	REPETITIONS
WORKOUT 1	Bench press	3	5–8
	Reverse grip lateral pull-downs	3	10–15
	Squats	3	5–8
	Leg curls	3	10–15
	Dumbbell shoulder press	3	5–8
	Incline curls	3	10–15
	Triceps press-downs	3	10–15

Training program 2

Intermediate three-day gym circuit program

	EXERCISES	SETS	REPETITIONS
WORKOUT 2	Incline dumbbell press	3	10–15
	Seated cable row	3	8–12
	Leg press	3	10–15
	Romanian deadlift	3	10–15
	Lateral raises	2	15–20
	Dumbbell hammer curl	2	15–20
	Overhead triceps extensions	2	10–15

Believe. Train. Nourish. Achieve.

Training program 2

Intermediate three-day gym circuit program

	EXERCISES	SETS	REPETITIONS
WORKOUT 3	Cable crossover	3	15–20
	Wide grip front lateral pull-downs	3	8–12
	Leg extensions	3	15–20
	Seated leg curls	3	10–15
	Cable face pulls	2	10–15
	Preacher curls	2	10–15
	Lying EZ bar extensions	2	10–15

Training program 3

Semi-advanced upper/lower four-day program

- Depending on your goals, try to do 6 to 12 repetitions per set.

- Sticking to the same rep range throughout the program will make it easier to monitor your progress.

- Increase reps and weights as you get fitter and/or as your goals require.

- Round each session off with your choice of abdominal and back-strengthening exercises to complement your workout.

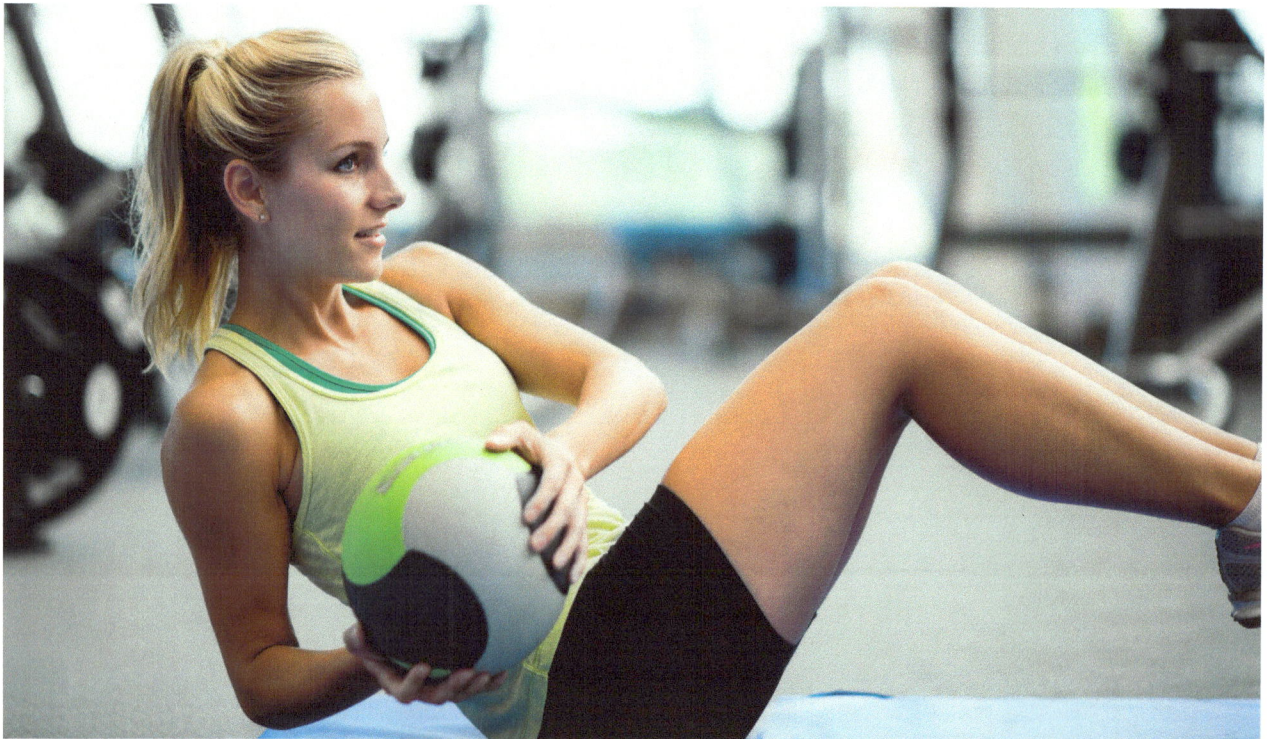

Semi-advanced upper/lower four-day program

Lower body workout (legs)

EXERCISES	SETS	REPETITIONS
Barbell squats	4	6–12
Bulgarian lunges	3	6–12
Leg press	4	6–12
Standing calf raises	4	6–12
Hamstring curls	4	6–12
Leg extensions	4	6–12
Planks, abs, and back extension exercises		5 minutes

WORKOUT 1

Training program 3

Semi-advanced upper/lower four-day program

Upper body workout (back and chest)

	EXERCISES	SETS	REPETITIONS
WORKOUT 2	Pull-ups	4	6–12
	Lateral pull-downs	4	6–12
	Machine rows	4	6–12
	Push-ups	4	6–12
	Bench press	4	6–12
	Pec flys	4	6–12
	Planks, abs, and back extension exercises		5 minutes

Believe. Train. Nourish. Achieve.

Training program 3

Semi-advanced upper/lower four-day program

Lower body workout (glutes)

	EXERCISES	SETS	REPETITIONS
WORKOUT 3	Hip thrusts	4	6–12
	Glute bridges	4	6–12
	Frog pumps	4	6–12
	Deadlifts	4	6–12
	Donkey kicks (weighted or banded)	4	6–12
	Fire hydrants (weighted or banded)	4	6–12
	Planks, abs, and back extension exercises		5 minutes

Training program 3

Semi-advanced upper/lower four-day program

Upper body workout (shoulders, biceps, triceps)

	EXERCISES	SETS	REPETITIONS
WORKOUT 4	Shoulder press	4	6–12
	Upright rows	4	6–12
	Front raises	3	6–12
	Lateral raises	3	6–12
	Rear deltoid flys	3	6–12
	Bicep curls	3	6–12
	Triceps rope pull-downs	3	6–12
	Planks, abs, and back extension exercises		5 minutes

Training program 4

Advanced complete split five-day program

This five-day advanced workout program includes the following workouts:

1. Chest and back

2. Legs and glutes

3. Chest, back, and shoulders

4. Legs, glutes, and arms

5. Legs, back, shoulders, and chest.

Please note:

- Warm-up sets are not included. We recommend using the warm-up exercises on page 120. Alternatively, you can use your own warm-up routine.

- As this is an advanced workout, keep the weights hard and heavy.

- That said, please train safely and effectively, and do not execute any exercises that are not suitable for you for any reason (e.g., injury). Instead, consult your trainer/coach/a fitness professional to find suitable alternatives.

- Always follow a cool-down program and stretch after each session.

- Specific abdominal exercises have not been included here as you will be working core muscles in all these workouts. However, you can add your own abdominal-specific exercises to the end of some of the workouts as desired.

Training program 4

Advanced complete split five-day program

Chest and back with optional abs

	EXERCISES	SETS	REPETITIONS
WORKOUT 1	Chest press	3	12
	Lateral pull-down	3	12
	Seated row	3	12
	Pec flys	3	12
	Lower back extensions (on mat)	3	12
	Push-ups	3	12
	Planks, abs, and back extension exercises (optional)		5 minutes

Training program 4

Advanced complete split five-day program

Legs and glutes

	EXERCISES	SETS	REPETITIONS
WORKOUT 2	Squats	3	12
	Hip thrusts	3	12
	Dumbbell lunges	3	12
	Leg extensions	3	12
	Leg curls	3	12
	Calf raises	3	15

Training program 4

Advanced complete split five-day program

Chest, back, and shoulders with optional abs

	EXERCISES	SETS	REPETITIONS
WORKOUT 3	Dumbbell shoulder press	3	12
	Dumbbell upright row	3	12
	Deltoid raise (alt front and side)	3	12
	Pectoral fly machine	3	12
	Rear deltoid seated fly machine	3	12
	Cable row	3	12
	Planks, abs, and back extension exercises (optional)		5 minutes

Believe. Train. Nourish. Achieve.

Training program 4

Advanced complete split five-day program

Legs, glutes, and arms

EXERCISES	SETS	REPETITIONS
Glute bridges	3	12
Inner thigh machine (adductor)	3	12
Outer thigh machine (abductor)	3	12
Hack squats	3	12
Cable bicep curls and tricep pull-down super set	3	12
Bicep curl machine	3	12

WORKOUT 4

Training program 4

Advanced complete split five-day program

Legs, back, shoulders, and chest

	EXERCISES	SETS	REPETITIONS
WORKOUT 5	Deadlifts	3	12
	Back extensions	3	12
	Shoulder press machine	3	12
	Bench press	3	12
	Assisted pull-up machine	3	12
	Bicep curl machine	3	12

Nourish

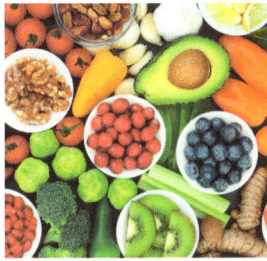

Mindful eating

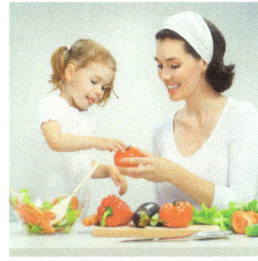

Balancing your diet
&
Macro- and micronutrients

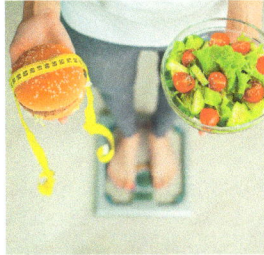

Eating for weight loss
&
Food tracking

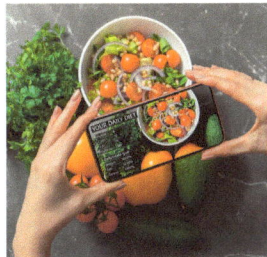

Hydration

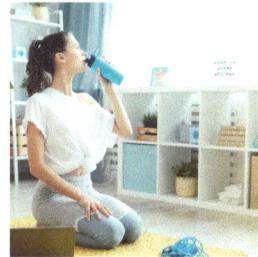

" One of the very nicest things about life is the way we must regularly stop whatever it is we are doing and devote our attention to eating.

Luciano Pavarotti

Food brings families, friends, even strangers, together. And, in doing so, provides nourishment not only to the body but also to the soul.

In Australia, we're surrounded by an abundance of readily available foods of all descriptions. From over-processed fast foods to highly nutritious organically grown fresh produce, it's all there for the taking. But along with the freedom to choose from such a huge selection of available food, comes the responsibility to choose wisely. That's where things get complicated.

Whether we're reaching for something to fill us up as we race from one appointment to the next or deciding on what to give the family for dinner, we tend to go for whatever's quickest, easiest, and cheapest, rather than spending time and effort selecting and preparing the most nutritious meals. And, with the many responsibilities that we juggle during our busy days, who can blame us for making food choices on the fly?

Since fast foods are so heavily marketed, they're almost always the first to come to mind when we're making snap choices about what to eat. We all know that lean protein and a garden salad makes a healthy meal, but it's going to be a hard sell when you're trying to feed your family on a cold winter's night.

The healthy food options in books and magazines may look delicious, but they are often also time-consuming, complicated, and require expensive, exotic ingredients that are unlikely to be used again. Celeriac? *Really?* And, if we are brave enough to try something new, it's very likely the kids won't even try it.

To make matters worse, many of us feel deeply conflicted about food because of long-term struggles to control body weight. We live in a nightmarish cycle consisting of periods where we virtually starve ourselves, followed by times when we overindulge, followed by guilt that only causes us to eat more and start the cycle all over again.

In this chapter, we're going to share some practical ways in which you can change your relationship with food from the love-hate struggle it so often becomes to one that's natural, easy, and enjoyable.

Once you have a good relationship with your food, you'll begin to enjoy eating simple healthy meals and experience all the benefits that come from eating a balanced diet.

Read on to discover how you can have more control over your weight, sleep better at night, enjoy a stronger immune system, and feel more energetic throughout the day.

Please consult a healthcare professional before following the advice in this book and/or beginning any new eating program to ensure that it is right for you.

NOTES

Believe. Train. Nourish. Achieve.

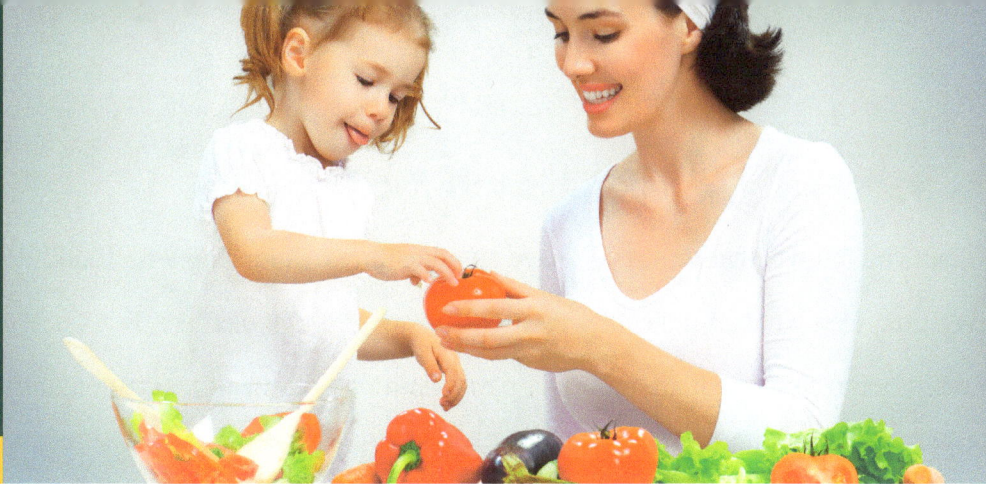

Mindful eating

Understanding our relationship to eating, cultivates a lot of insights
and helps us start living to our highest potential.

Natasa Pantovic

Animals eat to survive, but humans have more complex relationships with food. We don't just use it to fuel our bodies; we also eat for pleasure, comfort, and a host of other reasons. Whether we're socialising, mourning or celebrating, food is always there. In fact, food is an integral part of every aspect of our lives, cultures, and traditions. Yet, if we had to put a "relationship with food" status on social media, many of us would opt for "It's complicated." We love food, but we don't love the extra kilos, the high cholesterol, diabetes, and other health complaints that come with overeating and/or eating the so-called "bad" foods.

We're also well aware that telling ourselves certain foods and drinks are good or bad, allowed or not allowed, doesn't stop us from consuming them. In fact, it does the opposite. As soon as we impose rules on ourselves about which foods we can and cannot eat, we are inclined to rebel against those rules. We feel deprived of the restricted foods, and as a result, we binge on the food that's "off limits" seeing it as a treat.

What does an unhealthy relationship with food look like?

How can you tell whether or not you have an unhealthy relationship with food? Well, you probably have some idea what an unhealthy relationship with food looks like, but since getting your relationship with food right is such an important part of hitting your health, nutrition and weight loss goals, it's worth taking the time to unpack the concept a little here.

It's time for a change if your relationship with food involves any (or all) of the following:

- Feeling fear, guilt or shame about food or eating.

- Avoiding or restricting certain foods because you believe they are "bad".

- Having a long list of rules around the foods you can and cannot eat.

- *Obsessively* relying on calorie counters or diet apps to tell you when you must stop eating for the day. (Reasonable use of diet apps to achieve specific goals is fine. See Food Tracking chapter)

- Following extremely low-calorie diets (e.g., 900 calories or less per day) for extended periods.

- Ignoring legitimate hunger cues (e.g., feelings of weakness, fatigue or a grumbling stomach).

- Yo-yo dieting or fad dieting.

- Feeling stressed out and anxious when eating at restaurants and cafés because you're afraid of people judging your food choices.

- Binging on certain foods.

- Restricting your diet to a single type of food (e.g., only eating grapes, pineapple or grapefruit) to the exclusion of all other foods.

How to cultivate a healthy relationship with food

A healthy relationship with food starts with mindfully appreciating its many roles in your life and seeing it as more than just fuel for your body. When you do this, you'll be able to appreciate all foods in moderation, eat the foods that you enjoy without guilt and live a life that is neither defined nor controlled by food.

What does a healthy relationship with food look like?

When you have a healthy relationship with food, you:

- Give yourself permission to eat the foods you enjoy.
- Listen to and respect your natural and legitimate hunger cues.
- Eat to satisfy hunger and stop eating when you are full.
- Choose the foods that make you feel good and nourish your body.
- Regard all foods as equal without denying yourself any type of food.
- No longer obsess about weight.
- Don't pay attention to what others say about the foods you eat.
- Don't feel the need to justify food choices.
- Are no longer defined by your food choices.
- Eat all food in moderation.
- No longer focus solely on calories.

It's important not to be overwhelmed by this list. Bear in mind that transforming your relationship with food is not going to happen overnight. As is the case with other relationships, your relationship with food requires constant nurturing and long-term commitment.

Also, bear in mind that your relationship with food is not cast in stone and fixed for life. It will change and morph over time. Don't try to force yourself to get it right all at once and don't make it your goal to have a perfect relationship with food. That is impossible – we all have good days and bad days. Simply aim for more good days than bad. Tackle one aspect at a time. Go at your own pace, make small, lasting changes, and you will see results. Be patient and kind towards yourself along the way. And remember, it's about progress, not perfection.

How mindfulness can mend your relationship with food

We've said it before, and we'll say it again here: the benefits of daily mindfulness extend into every aspect of life. It should come as no surprise then that mindfulness is the key to building a better relationship with food.

> A good relationship with food has absolutely nothing to do with the quality of your diet or the types of food you eat, but rather how and why you choose the foods you eat.
>
> Katey Davidson, MScFN, RD, CPT

At the heart of a healthy relationship with food is the ability to make food choices that are no longer motivated by adherence to externally imposed rules or categories, and instead to choose foods based on how they make you feel and how they nourish your body.

Mindful eating empowers you by giving you unconditional permission to enjoy all foods equally, without guilt or shame. Rather than choosing your food based on other people's ideas of which foods are good or bad and feeling guilty when you eat certain foods, mindful eating teaches you to judge for yourself which foods you want to use to fuel your body.

As no foods are off-limits, you no longer feel deprived or restricted. You are free to choose, and you soon learn which foods offer the biggest benefits in terms of satisfaction, sustained energy, health, and immunity. Once you've identified them, choosing these foods over those that leave you feeling wrung-out, empty, and craving more becomes effortless.

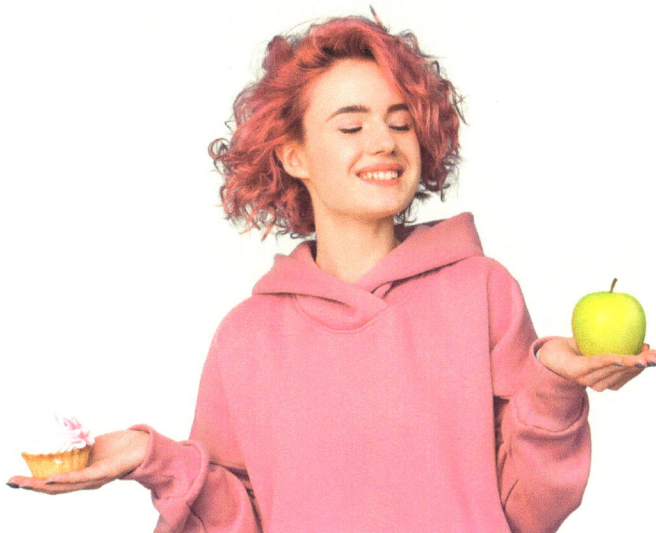

What is mindful eating?

Mindful eating is not about munching ruminatively on lettuce leaves and convincing yourself that they are delicious. It's not about striving for perfection in your diet, obsessively counting calories, fervently avoiding fast food or never allowing yourself a quick meal on the run. Instead, it's about focusing on food in a new way and being fully present as you shop for, prepare, serve, and eat your food.

Mindful eating helps curb the habit of binge eating to satisfy emotional needs (e.g., stress, sadness, anxiety, loneliness or boredom). When you eat mindfully, you're fully present for every bite.

Instead of rushing through meals in the car on the way to work, at your desk or in front of the TV, you're honouring your body by taking time out to nourish it. Savouring the taste, chewing your food properly, and enjoying the process of eating.

By maintaining an awareness of each moment while eating or drinking, observing how the food or drink makes you feel, and noticing the signals your body is sending about taste, texture, satisfaction, and fullness, mindful eating allows you to connect with your food and your body.

There is no judgement in this observation. Instead, there is acknowledgement and acceptance of the feelings and bodily sensations that you experience while you eat.

Through mindful eating, you become more in tune with your body and its needs. As a result, you learn to distinguish the subtle differences between the signals of hunger, thirst, and fullness.

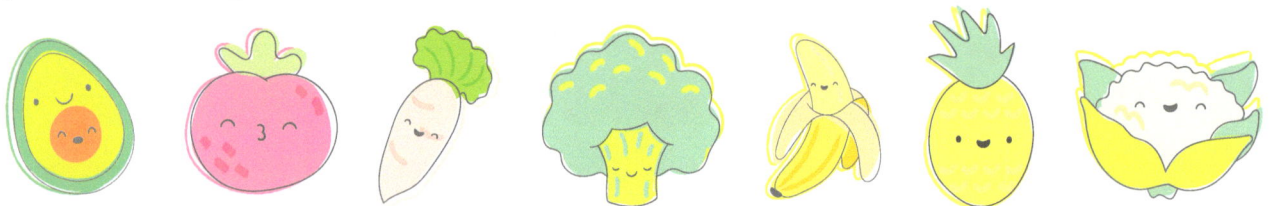

The benefits of mindful eating

It's hard to imagine how being mindful while you eat could lead to so many amazing health benefits. Yet, by simply sitting down, relaxing, and focusing on each and every bite, you'll be able to cultivate and maintain a healthy relationship with food and reap the rewards that come with it.

Here are just a few of the benefits of mindful eating

1. Improve your diet

By spending more time considering the foods you eat, how you prepare them, and how they make you feel – while you're eating them and afterwards – you will naturally begin to make better food choices. You may, for instance, notice that although a chocolate bar is great for picking you up during your 2:30 pm slump, it drops you again by 3 pm, and you're left wanting more. Switch the chocolate bar for a tub of yoghurt, and you'll notice how those peppy proteins keep you going for the rest of the afternoon. With results like these, next time you need a 2:30 pm pick-me-up, opting for the yoghurt will be a no-brainer.

2. Improve your relationship with food/drink

When you approach your meals more mindfully and question your motives for eating or drinking, you will notice the times when you're turning to food or drink for reasons other than hunger or thirst. For example, if you crack open a cold beer or pour a glass of vino every time you get in the door of an evening, chances are you're doing this more out of habit than out of the need to quench your thirst. Try substituting your wine or beer with soda water. Fancy it up with a twist of lime or lemon, and you'll not only break the habit but also keep your body well-hydrated.

3. Enjoy your food even more

Savouring every mouthful of food and focusing on taste, texture, aroma, and other sensations as you eat will help you fully experience all the different nuances of your food, and this will lead to greater enjoyment of your meals.

4. Improve digestion

You've probably been told (many times over) how important it is to chew your food properly. But how often do you really take the time to chew each bite? If you have a tendency to wolf down your meals on the go, you could end up with painful heartburn and indigestion.

With mindful eating, you slow down and chew each mouthful properly before swallowing. This aids digestion and helps you to feel better after your meals.

Besides reducing heartburn, chewing properly has very important health implications, particularly as studies indicate a rise in chronic digestive issues, such as gastro-oesophageal reflux disease (GERD), which are associated with poor eating habits. With symptoms including heartburn, persistent sore throat, chronic coughing, and, if left untreated, adult-onset asthma, ulcers, and precancerous lesions in the oesophagus, this unpleasant condition is not one you want to aggravate by neglecting to chew your food properly.

> " Mindful eating means simply eating or drinking while being aware of each bite or sip.
>
> Thích Nhất Hạnh

5. Break unhealthy eating habits

When you're eating mindfully, you'll also take the time to consider the types of food you're putting into your body. You'll be thinking about whether these foods will do you harm or nourish and strengthen your body. By selecting foods that will help you build a stronger, more resilient body, you'll naturally break unhealthy food addictions. And, by setting aside time for each meal, you'll be able to break past habits of eating on the run and settling for any food as long as it is fast and filling.

6. Feel fuller with less food

Focusing on your body's signals while you eat will help you to be more in tune with the effects of the foods you're eating and know when you've had enough.

By being more attentive and eating more slowly, you're allowing your body to keep track of what is coming in, which means it has time to tell you when it's full. Once you learn to recognise your body's cues, you'll discover that you feel full after eating much less food than your usual serving. This gives you plenty of time to stop eating when your body says it's had enough, effectively reducing the amount of overeating you're doing, which is great for weight control and overall health.

7. Manage food cravings

Mindful eating allows you to really get to know your body and its relationship with food. You'll be able to pick up on cravings and distinguish them from true hunger, making it easier to manage snacking and binge eating.

You'll also be able to make healthy substitutes when you do experience a craving. For example, eating a piece of fruit instead of a bag of lollies when you crave something sweet.

8. Maintain and even lose weight

Weight-loss experts will tell you that the secret to losing and maintaining a healthy weight is to keep a careful eye on what you put into your mouth. Mindful eating helps you to do this by shifting the focus from eating out of habit to eating for nourishment. When you practice mindful eating, you'll be making healthier food choices effortlessly, and you'll stop when you're full, all of which will help you to lose excess weight and keep it off.

9. Improve your mental health

Mindful eating helps to ease stress and anxiety by encouraging you to slow down during mealtimes. Taking a break from the chaos of your day to enjoy a meal gives you that much-needed escape from the stresses of the work day. It recharges your batteries, so you can think more clearly, solve problems with greater alacrity, and handle stressful situations with calm composure.

10. Make a deeper connection with your food

Mindful eating doesn't only occur while you're sitting down with the plate of food in front of you. It starts way before that, when you're planning your meals for the week and making your shopping list. Being mindful while you're selecting and shopping for food can help create a deeper understanding of where your food comes from, what it contains, how it's produced, and the journey it has taken to your plate.

Mindful food preparation is also important as it deepens your connection to the food you're about to eat. To get the full benefit of this practice, take your time preparing your meals, savouring the textures, aromas, and flavours of the ingredients as you add and prepare them.

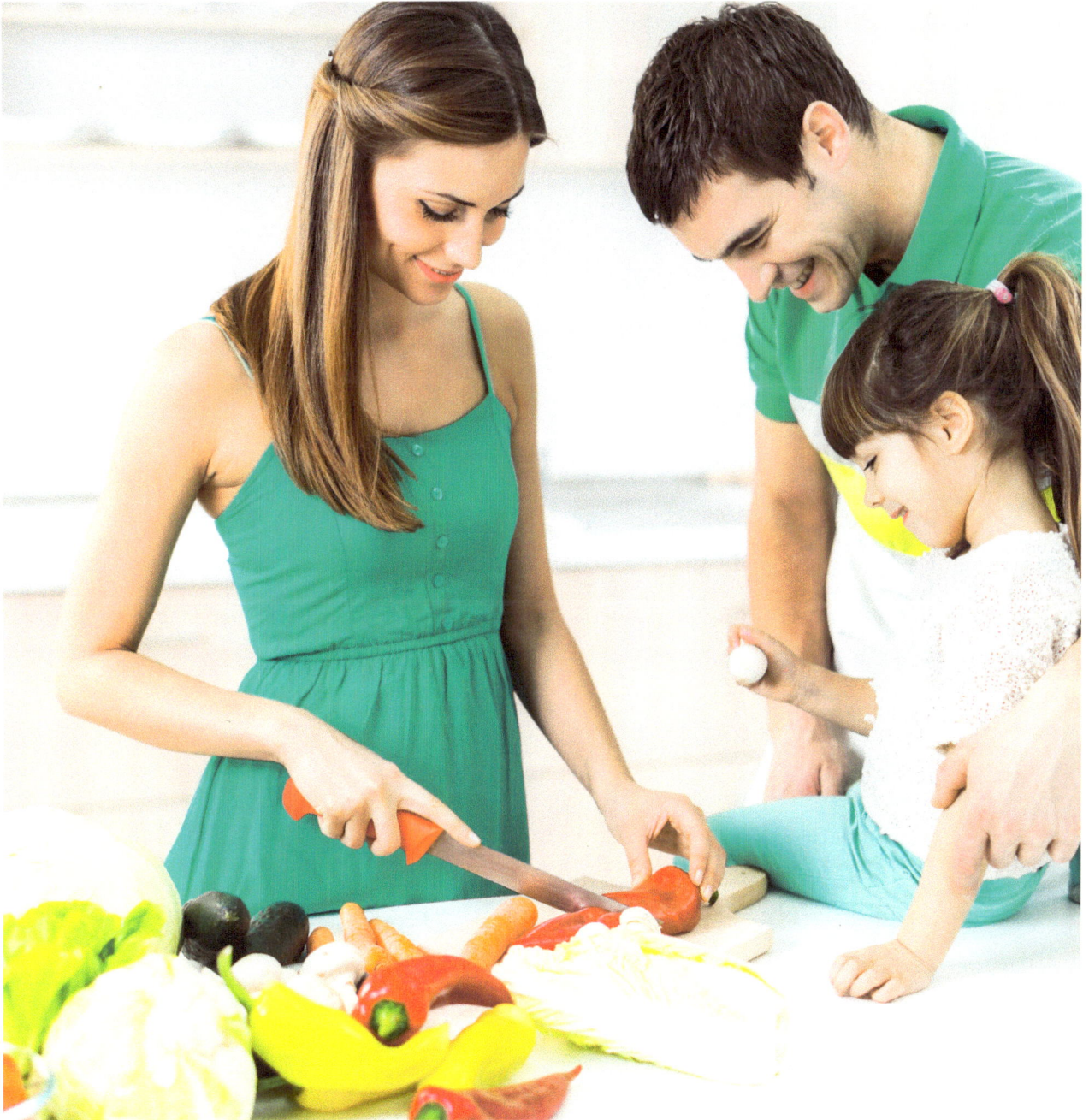

How to practice mindful eating

It's great to know that simply by paying attention while you eat, you can do so much for your health and wellbeing. But how exactly do you train yourself to be mindful about food?

It takes time and commitment to change the eating habits of a lifetime, and, if you've never done it before, it's going to take time to switch over to mindful eating.

Start small by simply focusing for five minutes during one meal a day and work your way up to being fully mindful every time you eat. Then concentrate on being mindful while making your shopping list, combing the aisles at your local supermarket, and preparing your meals at home.

Try to think carefully about your food choices, how you prepare each meal, and what your body is telling you while you're enjoying your meal. Whenever you notice your attention wavering, gently bring it back to your food. And yes, you can even eat mindfully at restaurants – simply focus on each item on the menu and make your selection with forethought and care, then take your time and relish every bite.

A step-by-step guide to mindful eating

1. Mindfully plan and prepare your meals

Mindful eating involves being fully present for every moment of every meal – from planning, purchase and preparation through to eating and washing up.

Mindfully planning your meals will help you to manage your hunger by eating at regular intervals throughout the day. It will also reduce the risk of raiding the fridge or pantry or grabbing take-out when you really would have preferred a proper meal, but were too hungry to wait while you prepared it. Try to plan your meals so that you arrive at the dinner table hungry but not starving from having skipped meals.

2. Dial in to your hunger

As you practice mindful eating, you will become more aware of how hungry you feel at different times of the day or night, and you will begin to question feelings of hunger that crop up at unexpected times.

When you find yourself wanting a snack between your regular mealtimes, ask whether you are truly hungry or whether you are actually bored, tired, trying to procrastinate, avoiding a task or satisfying a random craving. Make sure to only eat when you're truly hungry.

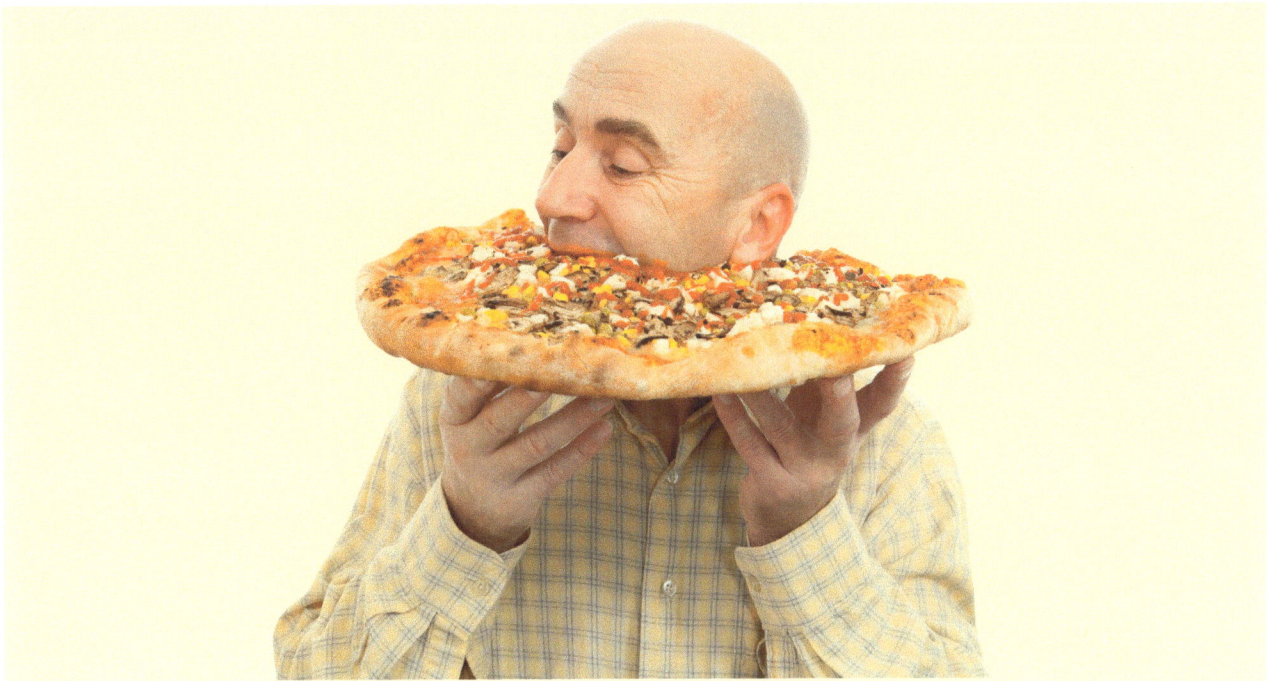

How to know if you're truly hungry

You can tell true physical hunger from false hunger (also called *hedonic hunger*) by paying attention to your body's hunger signals.

True physical hunger is your brain's way of telling you that you need to nourish your body. False or hedonic hunger, on the other hand, is the desire to eat for reasons other than the actual physical need for food. These reasons may include pleasure, habit, procrastination, satisfying a craving, overcoming boredom, and, oddly enough, thirst.

Physical hunger is easy to distinguish from hedonic hunger because it is accompanied by a rumbling stomach that communicates a real need for food. It pays to look out for this symptom when you're trying to decide whether you are truly hungry or just craving food. Try to only eat when you hear the rumbling.

If you have a nagging feeling of hunger without the rumbling, you may in fact be thirsty. To prevent dehydration in such cases, it's a good idea to drink a large glass of water and see what happens. If the hunger goes away, it was likely a thirst signal that the brain mistakenly broadcast as a hunger signal. Our brains often send out hunger signals when we're thirsty. We'll examine this in more detail in the Hydration section. In the meantime, let's get back to our Step-by-step guide...

3. Choose your surroundings carefully

Where possible, try to choose harmonious environment in which to eat. Move away from your desk or workspace and try to find a tranquil spot, free of distractions (e.g., phones, tablets, TVs, books or laptops) where you feel comfortable and at ease.

Once you've picked the ideal place to eat, take a moment to acknowledge your surroundings, but don't focus on them while you eat. Let them fade into the background and focus on your food.

4. Catch your breath

Take a few deep breaths until you feel calm, relaxed, and ready for your meal. Breathing deeply increases oxygen levels in your blood, which helps to improve your energy levels and gives you an overall sense of wellbeing.

It is easier to eat slowly and mindfully when you've taken time to unwind. Deep breathing has also been shown to placate hedonic hunger and relieve stress and anxiety associated with binge eating. Plus, relaxing before a meal aids digestion.

5. Take a moment to show gratitude before eating

Pausing for a moment in gratitude before you eat also helps you eat more mindfully. Even if you don't believe in giving thanks to a higher power, it's good to take a moment to reflect with gratitude on the fact that you are able to nourish your body in a world where nine million people die of hunger and related diseases every year (source: The World Counts: https://www.theworldcounts.com/challenges/people-and-poverty/hunger-and-obesity).

Your expression of gratitude does not have to take the form of a prayer. It can be done quietly – even wordlessly – but it should be done with deep sincerity. Ideally, it should be more meaningful than simply mouthing words that have been learned by rote. In it, you should appreciatively acknowledge where the food you're eating came from.

Express your gratitude for the plants and animals involved, the people who prepared it, and those who transported it to your door. Being more mindful of the origins of your food will also help you to make wiser, more sustainable food choices.

Try to maintain this attitude of gratitude towards your food not only while eating, but also throughout the whole process – from planning and selecting ingredients to preparing and enjoying your meal.

6. Focus on your food

Slow down and savour each bite – no matter what you are eating. Consider the food in front of you, paying particular attention to the aromas, colours, shapes, textures, and nourishment you'll be receiving from each item on your plate. By approaching food in this way, you'll get a much clearer picture of which foods you truly enjoy and how different foods affect your body. You'll also learn to read your body's fullness cues, so you won't overdo it.

7. Turn your thoughts and curiosity inwards

Pay attention to how you experience your meals, your eating habits, and your food. While you're eating, sit up straight and focus on your posture as well as on the signals your body is sending you about the food. Pay attention to how hot or cold your food is, how crunchy or soft, how it tastes, and how it makes you feel. This will help you uncover the reasons behind your food choices. You might even find yourself re-evaluating some choices, uncovering intolerances, and overcoming certain food addictions you thought you were stuck with.

Be curious about why you're eating and how your body is reacting to the food you're eating. Try to answer all or some of the following questions:

- Am I eating because I am hungry or because I'm bored, overwhelmed or procrastinating?
- If not hunger, what are my reasons for eating?
- Has this food solved the problem for me?
- Has this food satisfied my hunger/craving?
- How will this food make me feel mentally and physically – while I'm eating it and afterwards?
- What flavours am I tasting as I eat this?
- What textures can I feel?
- Is this enjoyable?
- Am I only eating this because it was available/cheap/easy?
- Is this food making me feel satisfied?
- How does this food affect me emotionally? Do I feel guilt, anger, shame, satisfaction or joy?

Start a food journal where you can write down your answers to these and other questions and observations regarding food and eating. This will allow you to discover the foods that satisfy and nourish you and those that cause negative reactions. Use these observations to guide your future food choices, so you get the maximum benefits both physically and emotionally from every meal.

NOTES

Believe. Train. Nourish. Achieve.

8. Get all your senses involved

Whether you're out shopping or at home cooking, serving, and eating, try to absorb every aspect of your food – textures, aromas, shapes, colours, and flavours. Take it all in. Focus on how each item (or bite) looks, smells, tastes, and feels.

When shopping, take your time, savour the scent of a ripe melon or enjoy the silky-smooth feeling of onion skin beneath your fingers.

When cooking, delight in the feeling of chopping up crisp fresh veggies or mashing potatoes. Relish the hiss of garlic as it hits the hot pan, and take pleasure in the lazy plop of stew in the slow cooker.

While eating, breathe in the rich aroma of minestrone soup, focus on the delicious combination of flavours in your salad or the crunch of a fresh carrot between your teeth.

While... Well, you get the idea.

9. Take a bite and chew thoroughly

Our grandparents told our parents, and they told us that we should chew each mouthful of food at least 32 times before swallowing. Yet, this is more than just an age-old adage, there are proven benefits to properly chewing your food. We'll discuss a few of them a little later on.

10. Notice how your food tastes and how it feels in your mouth

Imagine you're a judge on your favourite cooking show. Try to identify all the ingredients. Experience all the different flavours. Think about the texture of the food you're eating. How would you describe it? Is it crunchy, smooth, silky or springy?

11. Focus on the shift in your body as you eat

Notice how each food affects your body. Can you tell the moment when you have had enough? If you catch yourself rushing, remember to slow down. Take your time and stay focused on the present moment.

12. Lower your cutlery between bites

Pause between bites while eating. Put your cutlery down and take time to consider any feedback you're getting from your body. Are you feeling full yet? Are you satisfied? Do you still feel hungry? Or are you feeling bloated? Listen to your body and stop when you feel full. Pay attention to and be guided by the way your stomach feels rather than how much food is left on your plate. You can always keep the leftovers for later.

13. Share your meal times with friends and family

Don't just sit down and shovel food into your mouth. Make an occasion of mealtimes. Whenever possible, gather your family and friends around the table and enjoy your meals together. Their conversation will help you to eat more slowly and savour your food. While engaging with your loved ones, remember to pay attention to your body's signals of fullness and satiety and stay present while you eat.

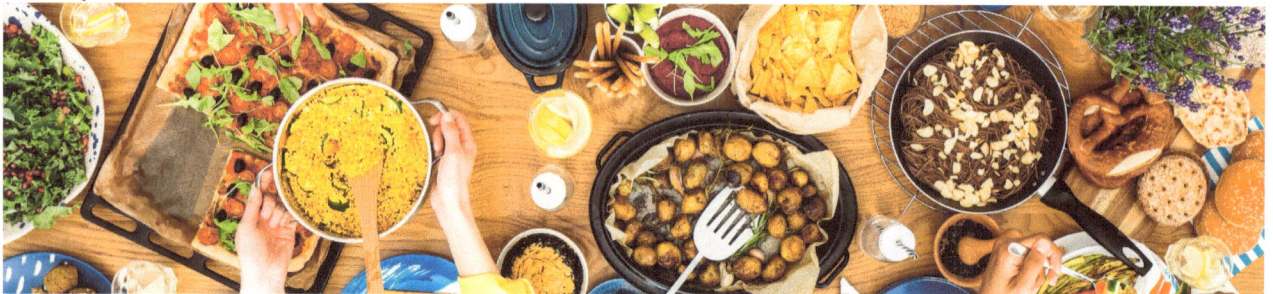

As promised, here are just a few of the benefits of chewing your food

1. Chewing helps break down food into smaller particles that are easier to digest.

2. Better digestion reduces the number of excess bacteria lingering in your intestines.

3. Chewing properly gives saliva a chance to work its magic on your food, breaking it down and allowing your stomach to absorb more nutrients and energy from the food.

4. Chewing helps release the hidden flavours in food, making it more enjoyable.

5. Chewing is good for your teeth. It stimulates saliva production, which helps keep teeth clean and reduces cavities.

6. Chewing makes it easier to maintain a healthy weight. Studies show that people who chewed more consumed fewer calories per day, lost weight more easily, lost fat, and claimed to be more energetic throughout the day.

A word of caution before you stock up on chewing gum

After hearing about the benefits of chewing, you might be tempted to rush out and stock up on gum. That's great, but you need to be careful in your choice of gum because it turns out that some types of chewing gum can be harmful to your teeth. Even sugar-free ones can cause acid build-up that results in cavities.

For best results, choose chewing gum that contains CPP-ACP. It's a remineralising agent derived from a milk protein called *casein phosphopeptide-amorphous calcium phosphate complex*. A 2008 clinical trial revealed that people using this type of gum not only had fewer newly developed tooth lesions (cavities) but also had a greater number of lesions that had regressed or remineralised.

Progress, not perfection

Don't let the idea of mindful eating become an obsession or another stress factor in your already stressful life. Remember you're aiming for progress, not perfection.

There is a place for mindfulness in your life, and there is also flexibility. Sometimes, you simply have to eat on the go. You may have a limited window in which to eat or go hungry for the rest of the day. In such cases, choose to nourish your body in whatever way you can. Try to choose the healthiest options from what is available to you at the time and don't beat yourself up about it.

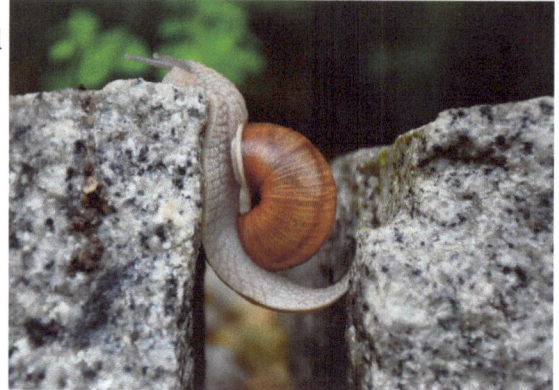

Just remember, you can still be mindful while eating fast food. Don't be tempted to multitask while you eat. Take a few deep breaths before you begin. Focus all your attention on your food (even if it is just for a few minutes). Pay attention to your body's signals and stop eating when you are full.

The most important thing is not to let one bad meal/day cause you to give up trying to eat well altogether. So, you ate takeaway for lunch today. No big deal. That doesn't mean you should give up on healthy eating and start eating this type of food every day. It *does* mean that you need to put that meal behind you and move on by making healthy food choices for your next meal, and the one after that, and so on.

Just like exercise, mindful eating takes practice. Every little bit you do each day counts. The more you practice slowing down and focusing on the eating process, the more satisfaction you'll find in eating. You'll fill up on less food and have greater control over your food choices and eating habits.

Don't struggle with this on your own

Remember, your relationship with food likely has a deep-rooted history, and it's not always possible to resolve without professional help. It's a good idea to reach out to a nutritionist, dietician, healthcare professional or therapist who can help you find the solutions you need to heal past hurts and mend your relationship with food.

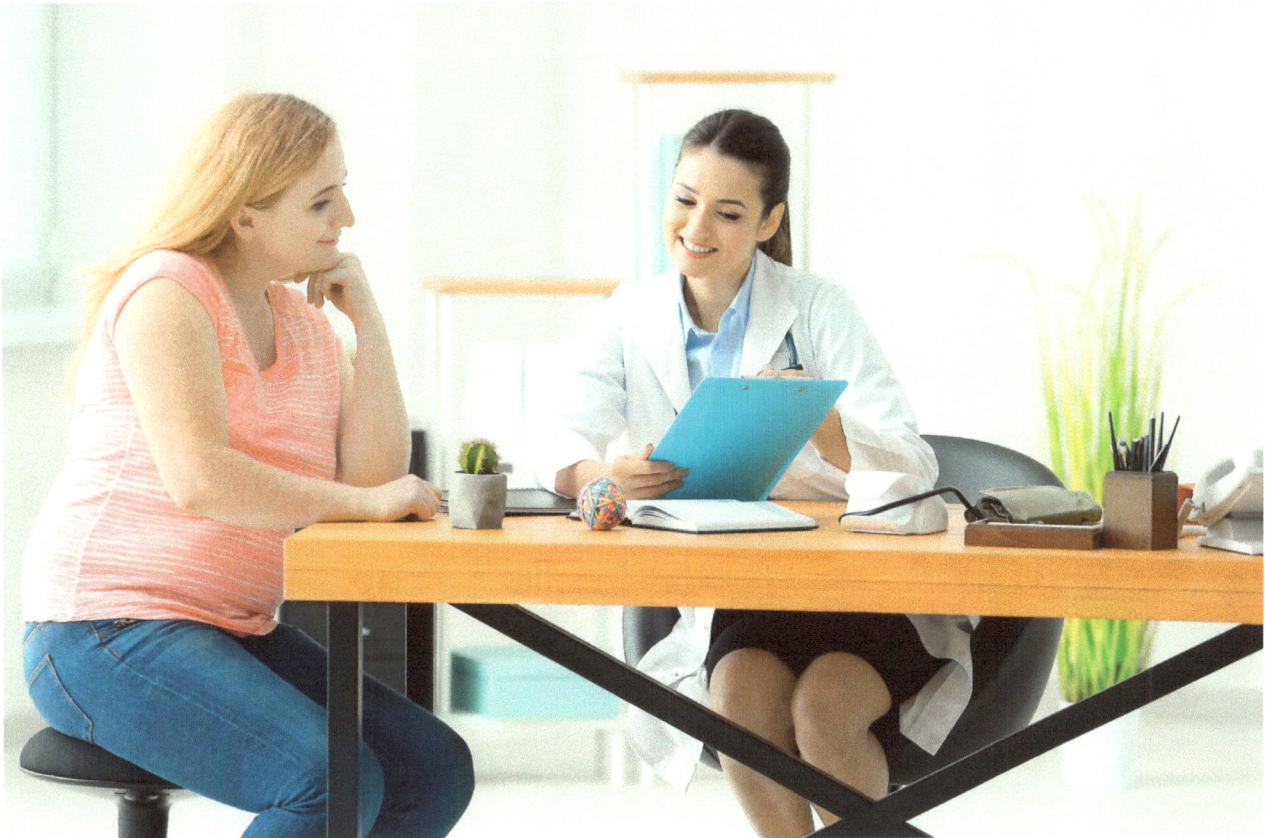

NOTES

Believe. Train. Nourish. Achieve.

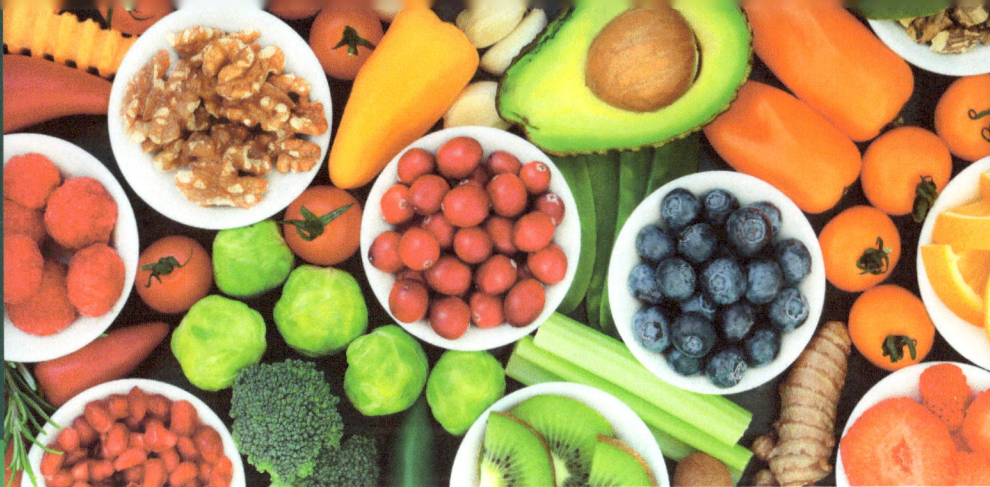

Balancing your diet

A healthy outside starts from the inside.
Robert Urich

It's safe to say that the search for the ideal diet has been going on for hundreds, if not thousands, of years. So, you'd think that by now we'd have a pretty good handle on what it takes to keep the human body performing at its peak. And, if we're honest, most of us *are* aware of the basic components of a balanced diet.

Remember the pie charts you created at school? (Hmm... pie) You know, the ones with segments for proteins, veggies, fruit, dairy, and grains? What about the much-touted CSIRO recommendations of five serves of veggies, two serves of fruit, one to three serves of protein, four to six serves of grain, and two to three serves of dairy per day? Sure, we've all seen these and yet, despite being aware of them, few people manage to put this knowledge into practice.

Part of the problem is that it's hard to visualise what *your* version of a balanced diet looks like. Or, for that matter, what a "serve" looks like. It's easier to just give up, feed our bodies whatever's handy and expect them to cope with what they get. Being the magnificent machines that they are, our bodies do the best they can to adapt and make the most of whatever we feed them.

But there's no way you can live your best life without properly nourishing your body. Eventually, you will pay the price for neglecting it. Years of not eating right can lead to chronic fatigue, illness, weakness, lack of mobility, mental health issues, and "silent killer" diseases, such as cancer, diabetes, and heart failure.

That said, it's never too late to start eating a well-balanced diet that will provide your body with the right amounts of energy and nutrients. A good diet will help you to recover, restore optimal bodily functions, achieve and maintain a healthy body weight, and reduce the risk of chronic disease.

In this chapter, we're going to examine exactly what we mean by a balanced diet, why your health and vitality depend on following this type of diet, and how you can use mindfulness to make food choices that support a balanced diet in your day-to-day life. Plus, we'll share some practical advice, so you can quickly tell whether or not you're getting your daily "serves" right.

What do we mean by a balanced diet, and why is it so important?

The short answer is that a balanced diet is one that provides your body with all the fuel and nutrients it needs to function properly.

Your diet must supply your body with a wide variety of nutrient-dense foods if you want it to carry out its many functions, including keeping you alive, helping you to move around, and supporting your brain as it tries to make sense of the world.

When it comes to creating a balanced diet and fuelling your body for success, it's important to make your food choices wisely. Being mindful when planning your daily meals will help to ensure that you include all the whole grains, fresh fruit and vegetables, lean protein, and dairy or unsweetened fortified dairy substitutes your body needs, in the right quantities.

What does a balanced diet really look like?

To stay healthy and thrive, your body needs a diet that includes a daily supply of:

- Vitamins
- Minerals
- Antioxidants
- Carbohydrates (including starches and fibre)
- Proteins
- Healthy fats.

The *Australian Guide to Healthy Eating* and *The Australian Dietary Guidelines* (www.eatforhealth.gov.au) explain exactly what's needed to keep your body happy and healthy. Let's take a closer look at their recommendations for a balanced diet.

Grain foods (one-third of daily intake)

Give refined white bread and bread rolls, sugary processed cereals, biscuits, and cakes the flick and fill one-third of your daily "plate" with natural wholegrain and/or high-fibre foods (e.g., whole oats, whole wheat, whole-grain rye, buckwheat, cracked wheat, millet, barley, spelt, quinoa, brown rice, corn, popcorn, whole-grain bread, whole-grain and whole-wheat pasta).

Why? Whole grain products deliver more vitamins, minerals, and fibre than their refined grain counterparts. Most of the nutrients contained in grains are found in the outer shell or hull, which is disposed of during the production of white flour. This process strips refined grain products of their nutritional value. Whole grain products, as the name suggests, include the entire grain (hull and all), retaining all their goodness.

There are huge health benefits associated with replacing refined grains with whole grains, not the least of which is the reduced risk of chronic diseases, including heart disease, type II diabetes, cancers, and more. Plus, whole grains add extra flavour and textures, making meals more enjoyable.

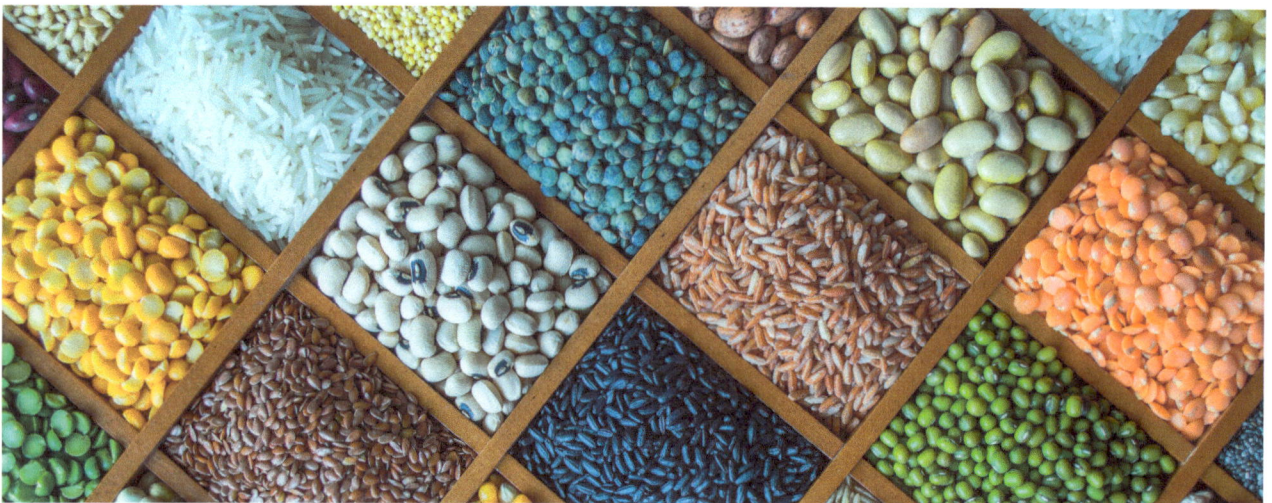

How many serves of grains is that and what does that look like?

The guidelines recommend that adults should eat four to six serves of grains per day, where one serve is approximately 500 kJ (120 Cal) or:

- One cupped handful (half a cup) of cooked grains, rice, pasta, noodles, barley, buckwheat, semolina, polenta, bulgur or quinoa
- Two-thirds of a cup of wheat cereal flakes
- A quarter cup of muesli
- Three multigrain crisp breads
- One wholemeal crumpet
- One small wholemeal or multigrain English muffin
- One slice of wholegrain bread.

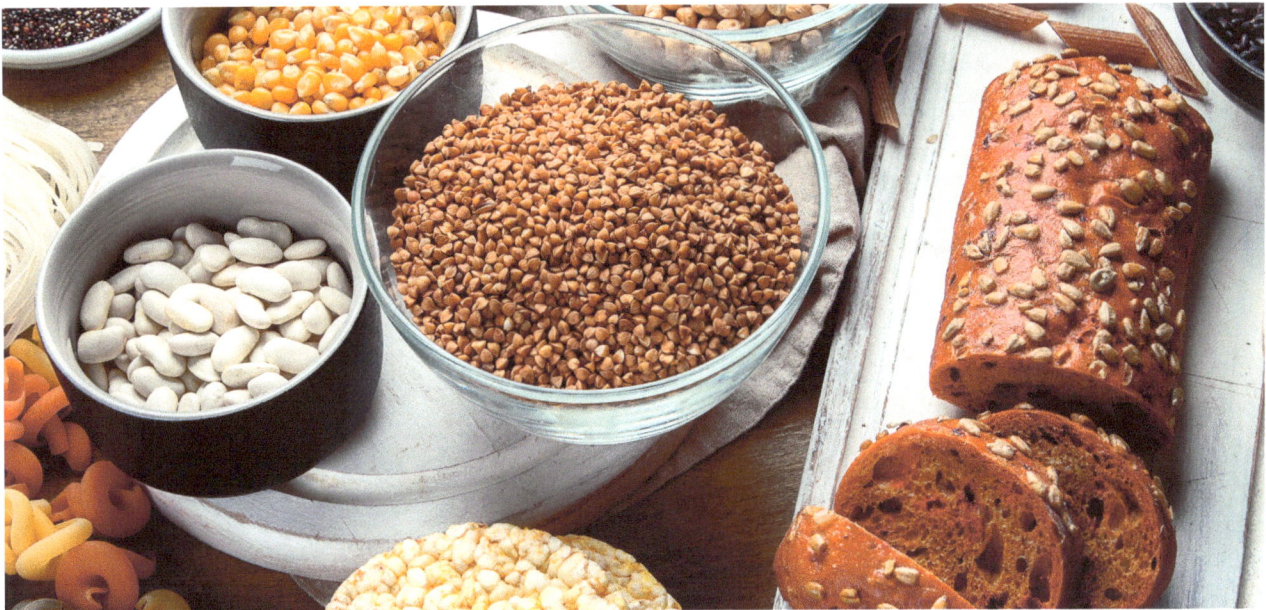

Oats-so-amazing

Oats have been shown to reduce cholesterol and are among the most nutrient-dense foods you can find. Not only are they a great source of carbohydrates and fibre (including the powerful beta-glucan fibre), but they also contain more protein and healthy fats than other grains. And they're loaded with vitamins, minerals, and antioxidants.

Eat just half a cup (78 g) of oats for breakfast, and you'll get

- Manganese: 191% of the recommended daily indication (RDI)
- Phosphorus: 41% of the RDI
- Magnesium: 34% of the RDI
- Copper: 24% of the RDI
- Iron: 20% of the RDI
- Zinc: 20% of the RDI
- Folate: 11% of the RDI
- Vitamin B1 (thiamine): 39% of the RDI
- Vitamin B5 (pantothenic acid): 10% of the RDI

    PLUS, calcium, potassium, vitamin B6 (pyridoxine), and vitamin B3 (niacin)

    PLUS, 51 g of carbs, 13 g protein, 5 g fat, and 8 g fibre.

    All neatly tied up and delivered with just 303 calories!

    You'll be hard-pressed to find a better nutritional deal anywhere else.

What's so special about beta-glucan fibre?

Well, beta-glucan fibre in oats has been shown to lower both total and LDL (bad) cholesterol, which are risk factors for heart disease. This means your morning bowl of oats will help to reduce your risk of heart disease – a leading cause of death globally.

Moreover, studies show that the antioxidants in oats work together with vitamin C to prevent LDL oxidation that produces inflammation of the arteries, damages tissues, and can raise the risk of heart attacks and strokes.

With all this goodness packed into a single grain, perhaps the question should be: can you afford NOT to have oats for brekkie?

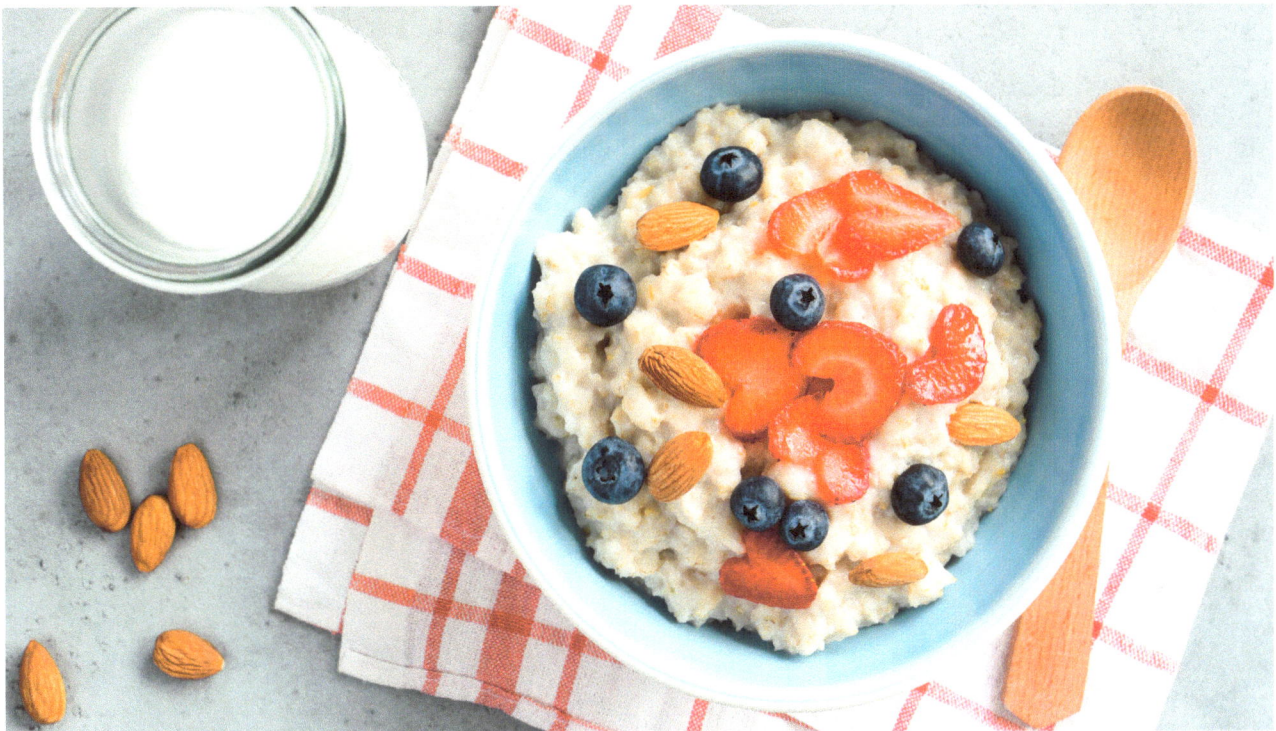

Fresh vegetables and legumes (one-third of daily intake)

One-third of your daily diet should be taken up by vegetables and legumes. These are key sources of essential vitamins, minerals, fibre, and antioxidants as well as healthy fats and oils.

They may not be the most popular of foods, but there are plenty of tasty ways to add more veggies to your diet, including smoothies, salads, dips/purees, soups, pasta dishes, roasted veggies or side dishes.

Select locally grown seasonal vegetables to get the best prices and highest nutritional value.

How many serves of vegetables and legumes is that and what does that look like?

The guidelines recommend that adults should eat five serves of vegetables and legumes per day, where one serve is approximately 75 g, 100–350 kJ (24–84 Cal) or:

- One handful (half a cup) of cooked vegetables
- One handful (half a cup) of cooked dried or canned beans, peas, lentils
- One fist-sized starchy vegetable (e.g., potato, sweet potato)
- One cup of green leafy vegetables or raw salad vegetables
- One medium tomato.

Eat the rainbow

Veggies are known for their great variety of colours, which indicate different nutrients.

To ensure you're getting all the nutrients you need, it's important to eat the entire rainbow of veggie colours. This includes a variety of items from each subcategory (green, red, purple, yellow, and orange, as well as legumes, peas, lentils, root veggies, etc.).

The dark leafy greens, such as spinach, kale, green beans, broccoli, collard greens, and Swiss chard, are most nutritious of all. So, be sure to include as many of these as possible.

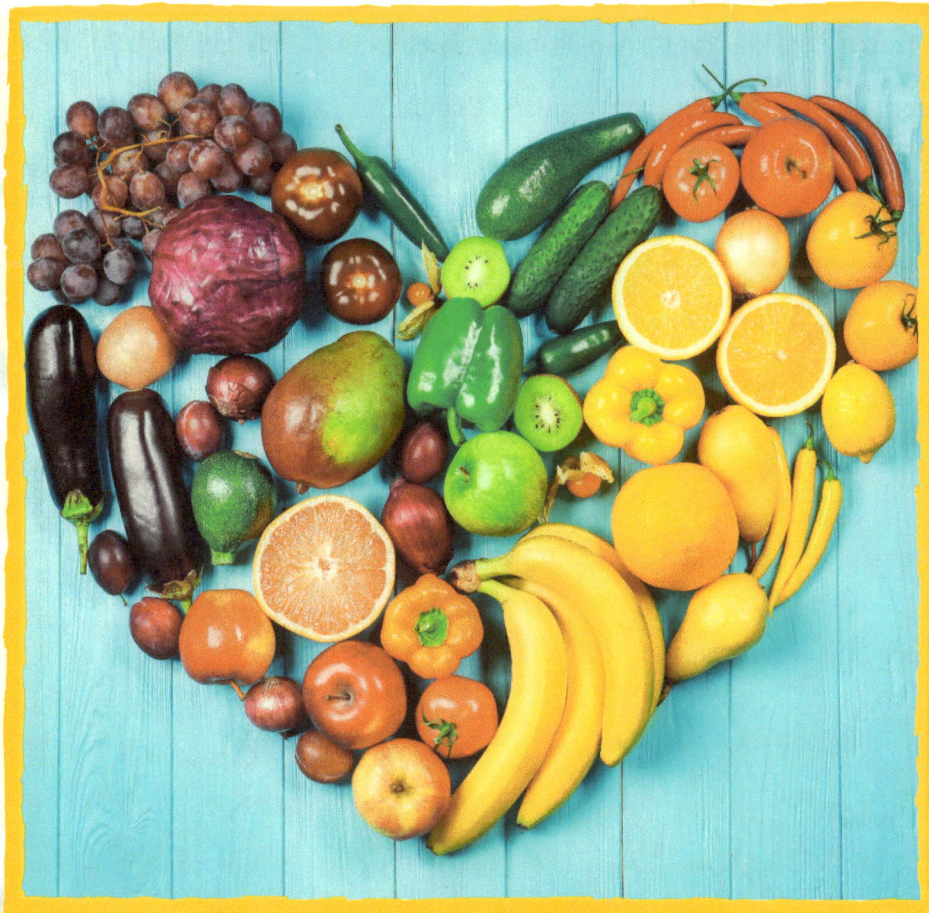

Fresh fruits (~10% of daily intake)

Approximately 10% of your daily food intake should ideally come from fresh fruit. As well as containing vitamins, minerals, and proteins, fruits are also high in fibre. Choose fresh fruits rather than dried or processed fruits to get the maximum fibre hit.

Berries (e.g., strawberries, raspberries, blackberries, and boysenberries) are bursting with fibre. Plus, they make a great addition to your whole-grain cereal or oatmeal in the morning. All that fibre will keep you feeling full and satisfied until lunchtime.

Fresh fruits are also great for satisfying a sweet tooth as they are packed with healthy natural sugars that offer a more sustained energy release than refined sugar. They also contain more nutrients than lollies, soft drinks or chocolates and are perfect as a quick snack or delicious dessert.

If you're craving something sweet that will keep you energised and satisfied for longer, choose fresh fruits such as apples, bananas oranges, peaches, and plums.

If you have diabetes or want to lose weight and/or prefer fruits that are low in sugar, stock up on raspberries (5 g per cup), strawberries (7 g per cup), grapefruit (9 g in one half of a medium-sized fruit), watermelon (10 g per cup), kiwi fruit (6 g per kiwi) or avocados (1 g per avo).

Be sure to choose local fruit that is in season. They are usually fresher and have a higher nutrient content.

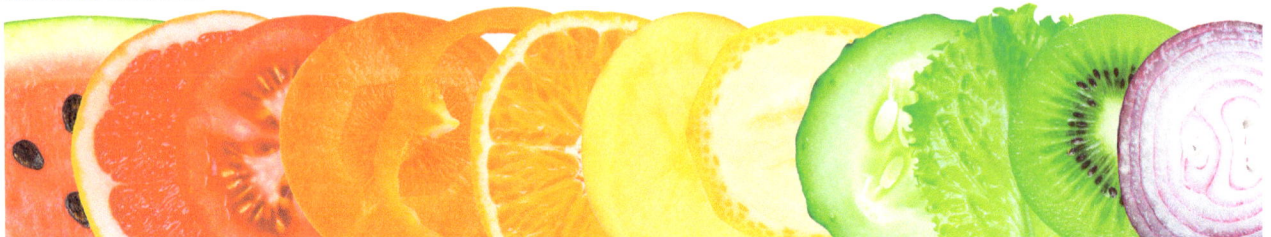

How many serves of fruit is that and what does that look like?

The guidelines recommend that adults should eat two serves of fruit per day where one serve is approximately 150 g, 350 kJ (84 Cal) or:

- One cupped handful of fruit pieces

- Two smaller-than-fist-sized fruit (apricots, kiwi fruits, plums)

- One cup of diced fruit

- One medium apple, orange, pear or banana.

Occasionally:

- 125ml (½ cup) fruit juice (no added sugar)

- 30 g dried fruit (e.g., four dried apricot halves, 1½ tablespoons of sultanas).

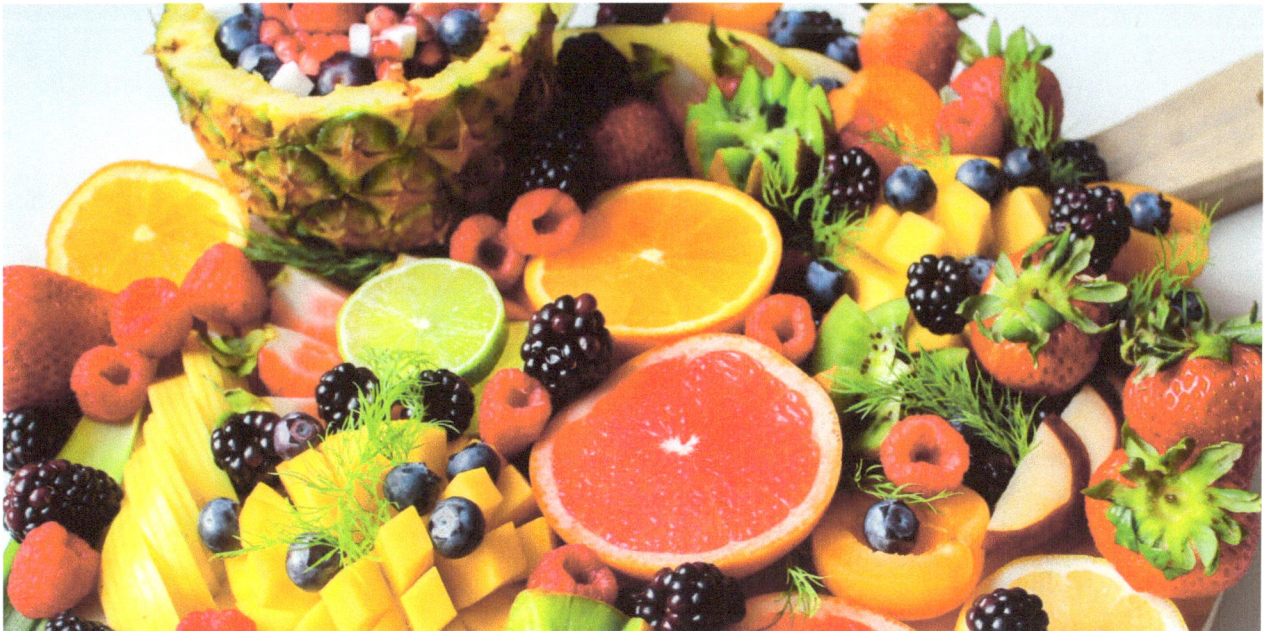

Life's better with a banana

Don't be deceived by fake news sites claiming that there is more sugar in a banana than there is in a donut. They are not comparing apples with apples. Admitedly, that fruit reference is a bit confusing, but what we mean is, that the sugar in bananas is natural and healthy, and totally not the same as the sugar in donuts. This means that the sugar you get from a banana won't cause a sugar spike and then drop you in a couple of minutes' time. Instead, it's backed by the protein, vitamins, and minerals in the banana. So, the banana will actually boost your body's nutrient levels and give you more energy for longer than any donut will. Plus, bananas contain none of the harmful trans-fats that donuts have in abundance.

Facts about fibre

Fibre is the name given to the parts of plants that provide strength and structure while the plant is alive and growing. Even though you can't digest fibre, it still plays an important role in your diet. In fact, it's vital for a healthy digestive system. Plus, because fibre is slow to pass through your system, fibre-rich foods have the benefit of helping you to feel full for longer. And, by slowing food down as it passes through your digestive tract, fibre allows you to absorb more nutrients and energy from your foods. This is why a high-fibre diet helps you to feel more energetic and healthier.

As a general rule, women need at least 25 g of fibre per day, whereas men need at least 38 g. The best way to reach these targets is to eat plenty of fresh fruit, veggies, and whole grains.

Dairy and/or unsweetened fortified dairy substitutes (~10% of daily intake)

Dairy and/or unsweetened fortified dairy substitutes should make up about 10% of your balanced diet. Dairy products provide essential nutrients including calcium, protein, and vitamin D.

If, however, you follow a vegan diet, dairy-free "milks" made from flaxseed, almonds, rice, coconut, soy or oats and fortified with calcium and other nutrients provide healthy alternatives to dairy. Choose unsweetened varieties to limit your intake of added sugars.

How many serves of dairy and/or unsweetened fortified dairy substitutes is that and what does that look like?

The guidelines recommend that adults should eat two serves of dairy and/or unsweetened fortified dairy substitutes per day, where one standard serve is about 500–600 kJ (120–144 Cal) or:

- Two slices (40 g) or a (4 x 3 x 2 cm) cube (40 g) of hard cheese (e.g., cheddar)
- Half a cup (120 g) of soft cheese (e.g., ricotta)
- One cup (250 ml) of milk
- One cup (250 ml) of soy, rice or other cereal drinks with at least 100 mg of added calcium per 100 ml
- Three-quarters of a cup (200 g) of yoghurt

The following foods contain the same amount of calcium as a serving of milk, yoghurt or cheese:

- One large handful (100 g) of almonds with skin
- One can (60 g) of sardines in water
- One half of a cup (100 g) of pink salmon with bones
- 100 g firm tofu (check the label to confirm calcium levels).

Protein, including lean meat, seafood, poultry, eggs, nuts, and seeds (~10% of daily intake)

Whether animal- or plant-based, the remaining 10% of your balanced diet should take the form of lean proteins.

If meat is an option for you, choose fresh, unprocessed poultry, beef, mutton or pork instead of processed meats as the latter are often high in sodium, contain preservatives, and have been linked to increased risk of cancer.

Meat, fish, and eggs are good sources of haem iron which combats fatigue and boosts the immune system. Beef and chicken livers and other organ meats are particularly rich sources of haem-iron, which is also found in abundance in oysters, clams, and mussels.

Fresh fish, including salmon, sardines, tuna, and other oily fish, are excellent sources of omega-6 and omega-3 fatty acids, which are essential for healthy cells.

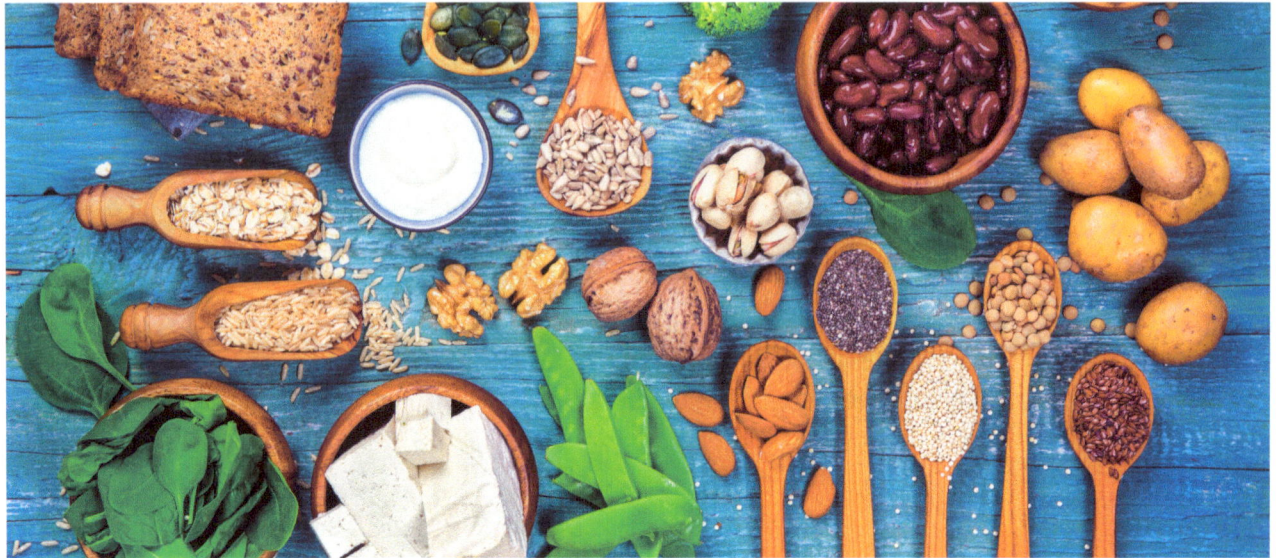

How many serves of protein is that and what does that look like?

The guidelines recommend that adults should eat two to three serves of protein per day where one standard serve is about 500–600 kJ (120–144 Cal) or:

- Two large (total of 120 g) eggs

- One cup (150 g) of cooked or canned legumes/beans, such as lentils, chickpeas or split peas (no added salt)

- 65 g of cooked (90–100 g raw) lean red meats, such as beef, lamb, veal, pork, goat or kangaroo

- 80 g of cooked (100 g raw) lean poultry, such as chicken or turkey

- 100 g of cooked (115 g raw) fish fillet or one small can (100g) of fish (salmon, mackerel or tuna)

- 170 g of tofu

- 30 g of nuts, seeds, peanut or almond butter, tahini, or other nut or seed paste (no added salt).

One man's meat is another man's tofu

Cultural, ethical, personal and religious ideologies influence the food choices we make, particularly when it comes to protein sources. For some, a balanced diet could include the full spectrum of animal and plant proteins, while for others, animal proteins may be limited or off the menu completely.

Pescatarians opt to include only seafood from the animal protein category, whereas some vegetarians limit their animal protein sources to eggs and dairy. Vegans consume no animal products at all and must supplement their protein intake with alternatives, such as beans, lentils, nuts, yeast flakes, tofu, tempeh, and/or soy-based products.

Whether you're a vegan, vegetarian, pescatarian or omnivore (i.e., you eat all types of food), it's important to include plant proteins in your diet. Try adding nuts and seeds to salads, nibbling on trail mix or a whole-nut bar at afternoon tea time, or grabbing a handful of almonds to snack on while you unwind in the evening.

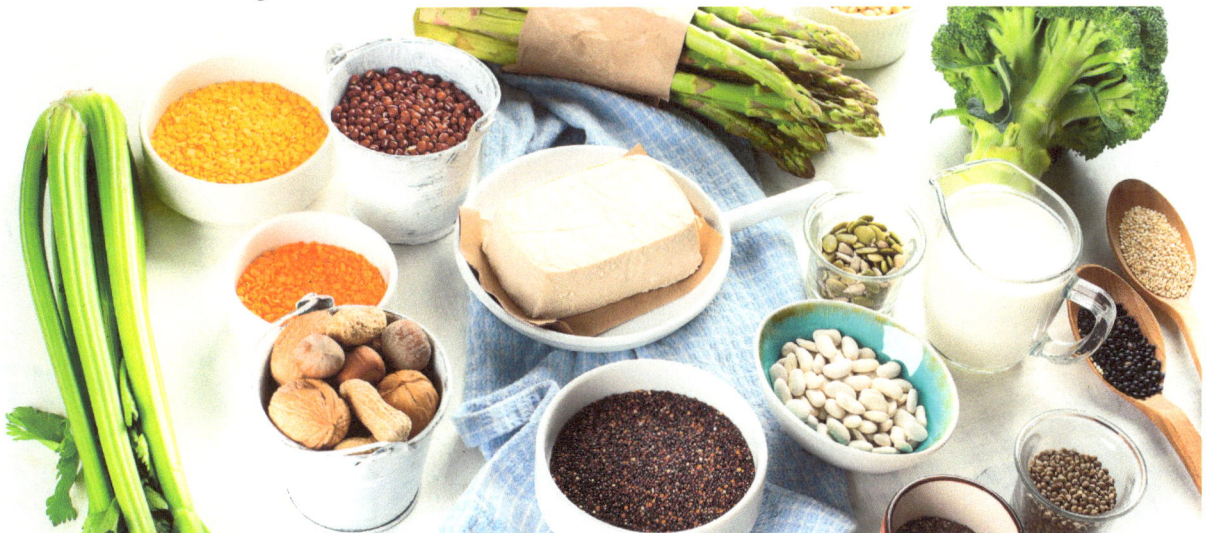

Foods to enjoy in limited amounts

As mentioned in the chapter on mindful eating, having a healthy relationship with food means giving yourself unconditional permission to choose the foods you want to eat. We explained that seeing foods as good or bad was part of the problem and not the solution to your food issues. In much the same way, denying yourself the occasional muffin, dessert or slice of cake will most likely only lead to bingeing on these foods later. This propels you into a spiral of guilt, depression, and frustration, which in turn leads to yo-yo dieting and poor nutrition.

A healthier approach is to allow yourself these foods in moderation and on special occasions without guilt or recrimination.

Examples of these "sometimes" foods include:

- Foods with high amounts of added sugar and salt
- Red and processed meats
- Highly processed foods
- Trans/unsaturated fats
- Refined grains
- Alcohol.

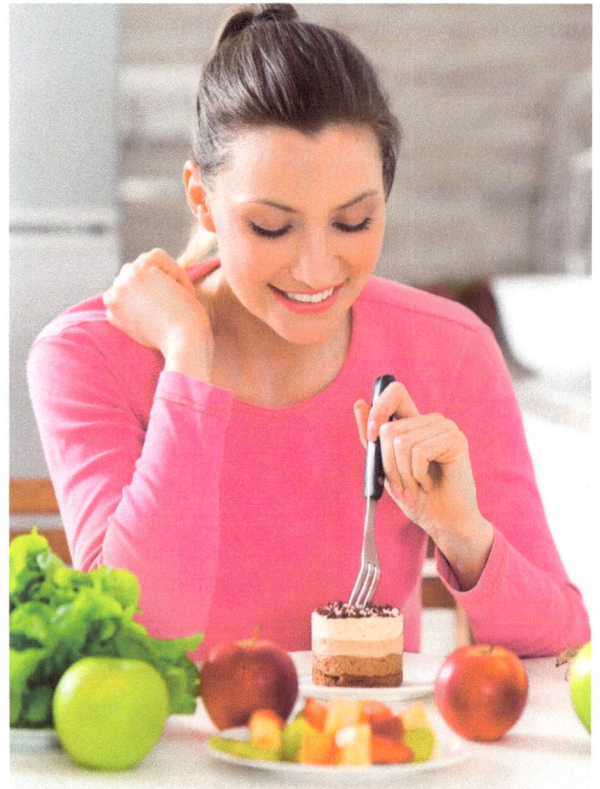

Facts about fats and oils

Fats and oils have a bad rap, but they are essential in small amounts for energy and healthy cells. Not all fats are needed in equal amounts, however. Unsaturated fats are best for the body. Saturated fats should be limited to less than 10% of the daily calorie intake, and trans fats should be avoided.

Extra virgin olive oil and fish oils get the tick of approval as they are high in *un*saturated fats, whereas butter, cheese, and heavy cream are high in saturated fats and should be consumed in limited amounts only. Trans fats are present in processed or pre-made foods, such as microwavable popcorn, fried fast foods, and bakery products, including muffins, cakes, pies, pastries, and donuts. Keep an eye out for the word "hydrogenated" in ingredient lists as this indicates the presence of trans fats.

Choose nutrient-dense foods over empty calories

When trying to decide which foods to include in your version of a balanced diet, it's important to consider the nutrient density of each food item and choose foods that contain high levels of nutrients, rather than those that contain loads of calories and very few nutrients.

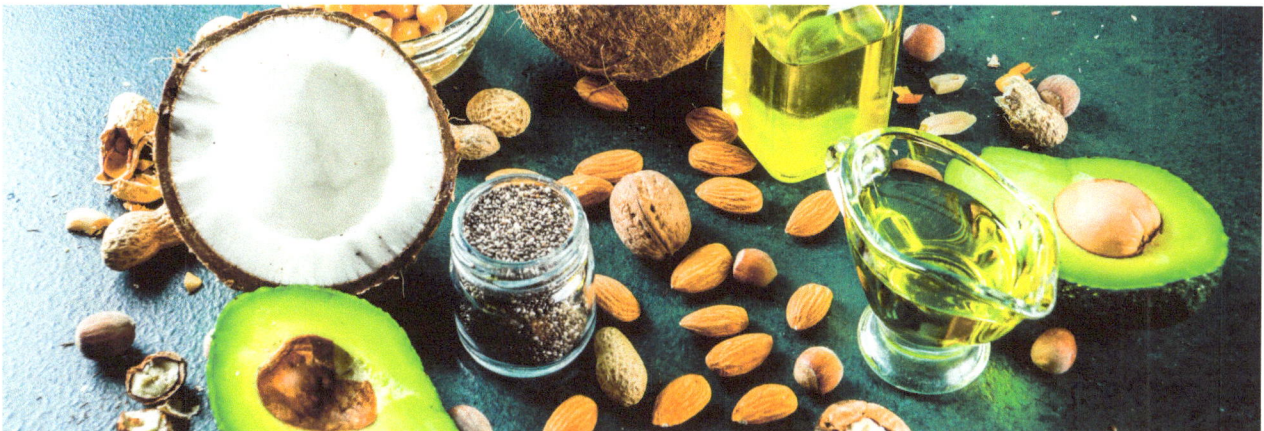

What are nutrient-dense foods, and how do we get them onto our plates?

Nutrient density refers to the number of nutrients in a food relative to the calories it delivers.

When looking for nutrient-dense foods, seek out natural, unprocessed, whole organic foods that are not manmade, have not been chemically altered, and do not contain any synthetic ingredients.

A good rule of thumb is to choose unpackaged foods, such as fresh meats, fruits, and vegetables, and limit packaged foods to those with fewer than four ingredients. Avoid foods with unpronounceable ingredients in their ingredient lists.

What are the benefits of nutrient-dense foods?

1. More nutrients per calorie

With nutrient-dense foods, you're getting more nutrients per calorie. So, you get a higher amount of nutrients and feel more satisfied for longer. *#winnng*

2. A wider variety of food choices

When you're selecting your foods based on nutrient density, you're not restricting yourself to the so-called "rabbit food" that we always think of when we think about a healthy diet. With this approach, salads are not the *only* stars of the show. Instead, you have a whole range of delicious foods, which fit the nutrient-dense criterion, to add to your daily meal plan. These include fish, lean red meat, eggs, beans, peas, raw nuts and seeds, poultry, and whole grains.

3. Eat more for fewer calories

Because nutrient-dense foods contain more fibre and water, and no added sugars, you will be able to consume more food, while staying within your daily calorie allowance, and you may even lose weight in the process.

When you're eating a lot of nutrient-dense foods, like veggies and fruit, and moderate amounts of legumes and grains, you'll also end up feeling fuller and be less likely to overeat.

4. Feel fuller for longer

Imagine swapping your daily bowl of sugary cereal with delicious free-range eggs on toast. Yummy and filling. Each large egg has a low calorie count of just 75 calories and contains plenty of B-vitamins, choline, vitamin D, healthy omega-3 fats, and protein. And, there's no added sugar. Plus, if you boil them and use a healthy spread, there are no saturated fats either. So, by simply choosing the more nutrient-dense option, instead of getting a huge sugar rush that drops you like a sack of potatoes half an hour later, you'll feel more satisfied and fuller for longer, and you'll be better able to cope with your day.

5. Get the essential macro- and micronutrients your body needs

Your body requires both macro- and micronutrients to function properly. We'll go into more detail about these in the next chapter, but for now, it's important to note that nutrient-dense foods provide micronutrients, such as essential vitamins, trace minerals, and electrolytes (e.g., magnesium, calcium, and potassium), as well as macronutrients, including simple and complex carbohydrates, proteins (amino acids), and a range of healthy fats.

6. Increased fibre gives digestion the green light

By choosing nutrient-dense whole foods, you'll naturally increase your fibre intake, which, in addition to keeping you satisfied, promotes healthy weight loss/management and helps to prevent diseases of the digestive system.

7. Prevent cancers and chronic illnesses

Nutrient-dense foods act as natural anti-inflammatory agents, reducing inflammation in the body, which helps prevent certain types of cancer and chronic illnesses, such as diabetes and heart disease. These foods also contain antioxidants and phytochemicals that cannot be replicated in synthetic supplements, and which support the immune system, helping your body to ward off infections, detoxify, and repair cells.

8. Effortlessly achieve and maintain a healthy body weight

When you're prioritising nutrient-dense foods, it becomes much easier to eat only the optimal amounts of calories each day, without restricting yourself to extremely low-calorie diets.

Simply reduce or remove the number of "empty calories" you consume by removing highly processed foods from your diet and replacing them with nutrient-dense calories from more satisfying whole foods.

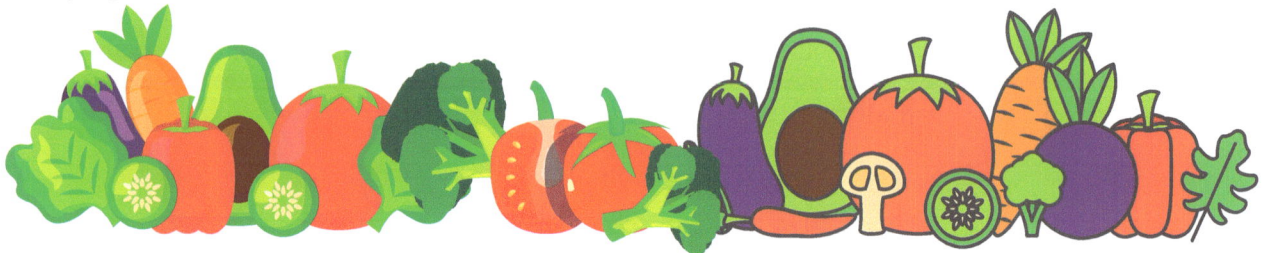

What's good for the goose may not be good for the gander

Another important aspect to consider when working out what your version of a balanced diet will look like is whether your body can cope with certain foods. A multigrain sandwich may be a healthy lunch option in many a balanced diet. However, that same sandwich would be no good for someone who is gluten intolerant.

Certain fruits that are high in sugar may not be suitable as part of a healthy diet for people living with diabetes. It's important to know your food triggers and intolerances and replace these foods with alternatives that will leave you feeling healthy and happy.

Talk to the experts

If you have (or suspect that you might have) food intolerances, health issues, such as coeliac disease or diabetes, or specific dietary requirements (e.g., prenatal, breastfeeding, vegan or athletic nutrition), please reach out to a professional dietician who will help you to find the ideal balanced diet to suit your needs.

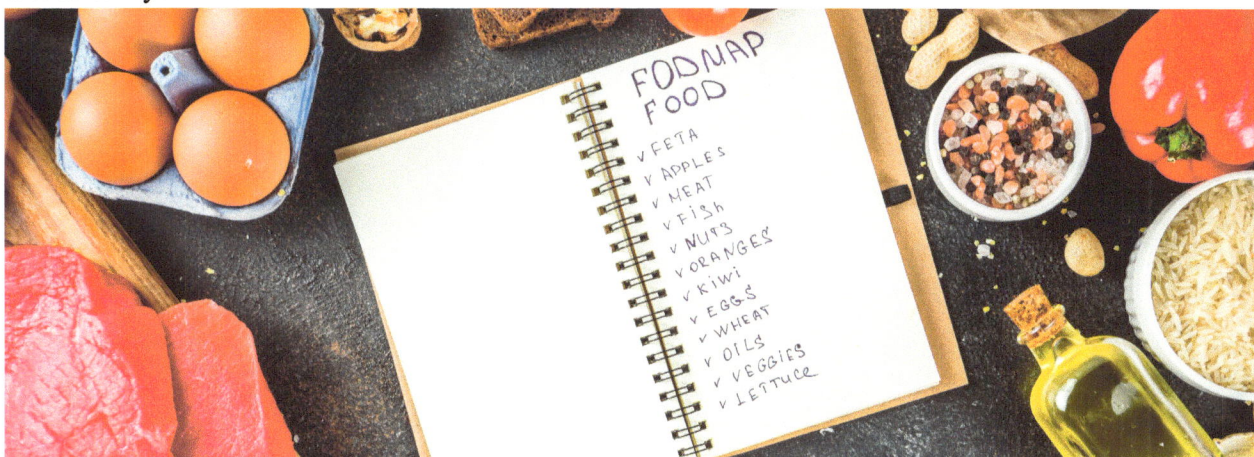

NOTES

Believe. Train. Nourish. Achieve.

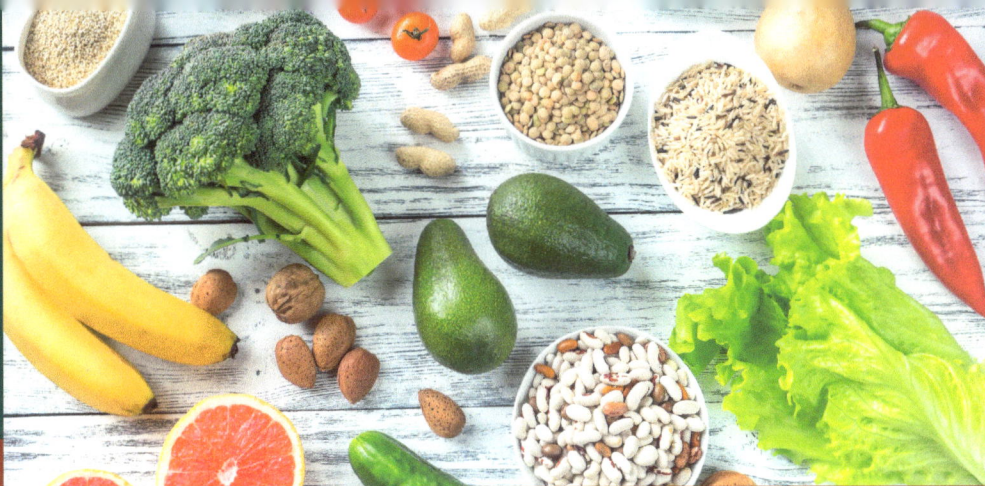

Macro- and micronutrients

We need macronutrients to help with energy and we need micronutrients to help our bodies to be healthy and digest those macronutrients.
Dr Donald Hensrud

In this chapter, we're going to take a closer look at nutrients and the specific roles they perform in your body. We'll share which foods are the best sources of these important nutrients, so it's easy for you to make wise food choices as you build your version of a healthy balanced diet.

If you've ever heard athletic types talking about macro- and micronutrients, and wondered what they're really on about, this chapter has the answers you've been looking for. Read on and, next time Ken and Barb are going on about "balancing our macros", you'll be able to surprise them with some insightful comments of your own.

Macro- and micronutrients work together to provide your body with the energy and nourishment it needs to function properly and ward off illness. Put simply, macronutrients provide you with energy, and micronutrients support cell functioning. Let's examine them in more detail.

Macronutrients

Macronutrients (affectionately known as macros) include carbohydrates, fats, and proteins. They make up the three main sources of energy in your diet. These little beauties help your body to grow and function properly. Your body cannot produce them on its own, which is why they need to be included, in healthy amounts, in your balanced meal plan. All macronutrients provide your body with energy, but each type fulfills a unique and specific function.

Carbohydrates

This group of macros includes the sugars, starches, and fibre that are found in fresh fruit, vegetables, and grains. Carbohydrates (carbs) provide approximately four calories per gram of ready energy to the body. They are easily broken down into glucose, which is used to fuel cells in the muscles and brain. There are two varieties of carbohydrates out there, and one type is a better energy source than the other.

Simple carbohydrates are those high-calorie, low-nutrient carbs found in baked goods, refined flour, corn syrup, and white sugar. They are low in fibre and high in saturated fats. They're rapidly digested, give you a massive energy hit really fast and then drop you as fast as the world's highest and fastest drop tower amusement ride (where riders reach speeds of 140 km/hr). Well, maybe not *that* fast, but you get the idea.

Complex carbohydrates are your typical nutrient-dense foods – they're processed more slowly and are packed with nutrients. They're also low in saturated fats, naturally high in fibre, and free from refined sugars or grains.

And, just when you thought they couldn't get any better, foods containing complex carbs are also usually lower in calories than foods containing simple carbs.

There are a variety of reasons why you might choose to follow low- or no-carb diets, but if carbs are an option for you, your body will thank you for choosing complex carbohydrates over simple carbs.

Good sources of complex carbohydrates include fresh fruit and vegetables, whole grains (e.g., brown rice, wholewheat/multigrain bread, wholewheat pasta) and legumes (e.g., all types of beans, peas, lentils and chickpeas).

Proteins

Proteins deliver approximately four calories of energy per gram, and they are a source of essential amino acids, which are the building blocks of the body. Each protein contains different types and arrangements of amino acids.

Proteins are used to produce hormones, enzymes, and antibodies as well as being integral to certain bodily structures such as connective tissue, skin, hair, and muscle fibres.

The recommended daily protein intake for moderately active adults is between 0.75 g and 1 g of protein per kilogram of body weight. Athletes, bodybuilders, and those wanting to increase muscle mass may require more protein per kilogram and should consult a nutritionist to determine the optimal amounts of proteins and other macros required to meet their goals.

Proteins can be derived from animal and/or plant-based sources. However, only animal protein sources (meat, eggs, poultry, and fish) contain all the essential amino acids required by the human body. Proteins from plants, including soy products, tofu, quinoa, leafy greens, nuts, and seeds, each lack at least one essential amino acid. To combat this deficiency, it's vital that vegans and vegetarians include a wide variety of plant protein sources in their daily diets.

Fats

The third type of macronutrient that your body requires is fat. Despite their dodgy reputation, you *do* need them. Just like carbohydrates and proteins, fats provide energy, and they pack a powerful punch with a whopping nine calories per gram.

Broadly, there are two types of fats – saturated and unsaturated fats. Strictly speaking, your body only needs unsaturated fats, although saturated fats do have some value – they supplement the body's natural supply of cholesterol, which plays an important role in hormone production. That said, your body is quite capable of producing its own cholesterol. And you're really no worse off without saturated fats. In fact, too much cholesterol can increase your risk of heart disease. So, regardless of their contribution, you should limit saturated fats as much as possible.

As a rule, total fats should make up 30% to 35% of your daily calorie budget with saturated fats taking up less than 10%.

Fish (especially fatty fish, such as mackerel, sardines, tuna, and salmon), and plant-based produce (e.g., avocados, nuts, olive oil, flaxseed oil, canola oil, and chia seeds) are good sources of unsaturated fats. Sources of saturated fats include animal fats, butter, whole milk, and coconut oil.

Trans fats, also known as trans-unsaturated fatty acids, are a type of unsaturated fat that should be avoided as much as possible. Although they are present in small amounts in milk and meat, these fats are most commonly found in fried fast foods, fried fast foods, highly processed or pre-made foods (e.g., microwavable popcorn), and bakery products (tarts, cakes, pies, pastries, and slices). Remember to watch out for and avoid foods with the word "hydrogenated" in their ingredient lists.

Balancing your macros

Tracking and balancing your macros provides an alternative approach to calorie counting when it comes to maintaining a balanced diet and achieving weight loss.

By focusing on your intake of fats, proteins, and carbs, you can choose from a wider range of foods than if you stick to just counting calories. Some macro-based nutrition plans even go so far as to offer followers the flexibility to choose whichever foods they like, as long as they fit into their allocation of macros for the day. Hence, this method has a reputation for being less restrictive than traditional calorie-counting.

We'll discuss how to calculate and track your macros for weight loss in greater detail in the Eating for Weight Loss chapter. For now, it's enough to know that as a general rule, the acceptable macronutrient distribution ranges (AMDR) for a healthy balanced diet are 45% to 65% of your daily calories from carbs, 20% to 35% from fats, and 10% to 35% from protein.

Some popular nutrition apps default for convenience to 50% carbohydrates, 20% protein, and 30% fat, while allowing users to adjusted these values according to their unique requirements.

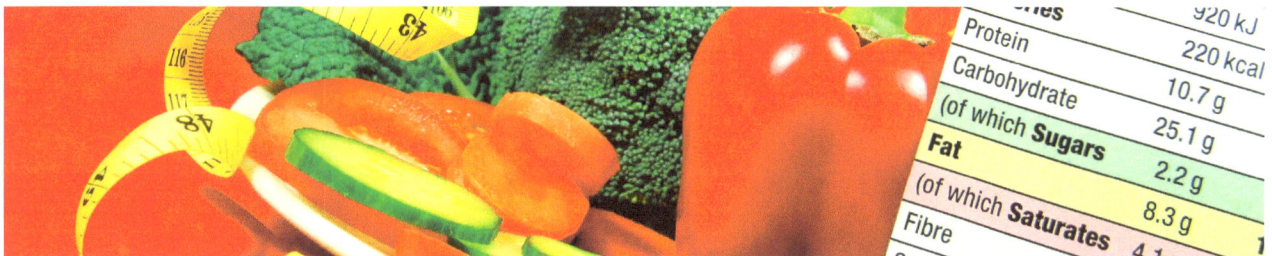

Not all macros are created equal

Macro tracking is about more than just adding up all the carbs, proteins, and fats you're consuming. The source of your macros is just as important for your overall health.

Some foods contain more of one macro than others, so it pays to include a variety of foods in your diet. For example, most pasta, cereals, rice, bread, legumes, fruit, and veggies are high in carbohydrates and low in fats and proteins, whereas nuts, seeds, olives, and cheese are high in fat and lower in carbohydrates. Avocados, olive oil, and coconut milk are high in fats, and low in proteins, whereas Greek yoghurt, cottage or cream cheese, poultry, beef, and whey protein powder are all high in protein and lower in fat. Eggs, meat, and fish are high in protein and low in carbohydrates. Phew! Good thing we have apps to keep track of all this for us.

To make things just that little bit more complicated, some foods contain the same amount of a particular macro but differ in the micronutrients that they deliver to the body. This is one of the weaknesses of some macro-based diets – they don't take micronutrients into account.

We'll look at micronutrients in a second, but first, let's round up our discussion of macros with a few things to bear in mind when planning your macro intake.

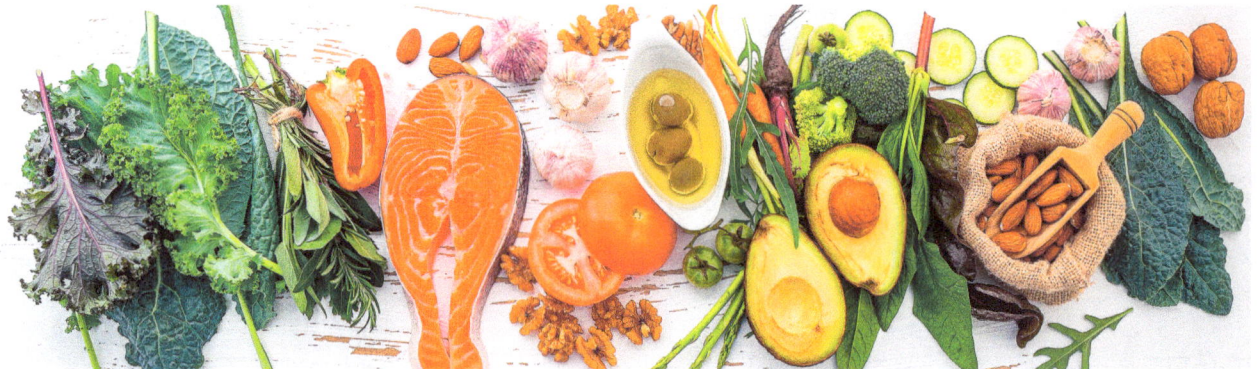

Things to consider when balancing your macros

1. Focus on maintaining a healthy balanced diet that will lead to long-term weight loss, rather than opting to starve your body of essential nourishment. The latter may lead to rapid weight loss initially, but it's not sustainable. You'll only end up feeling sick and will likely rebound putting on more weight than you lost.

2. Choose complex carbohydrates over refined carbs. Foods such as fresh fruit, veggies, and whole grains will moderate your blood sugar levels and keep you feeling full for longer.

3. Limit refined carbs to small quantities on special occasions.

4. Increase your intake of lean proteins that promote muscle repair and growth without the heavy calorie load of fats or carbs.

5. Fats have an important role to play in keeping you feeling full and promoting brain health, so don't skimp on healthy fats found in foods rich in omega-3s and omega-6s, such as avocados, nuts, and fatty fish.

6. Always consult your doctor or dietician before making changes to your diet, particularly if you have diabetes, kidney disease or other digestion-related symptoms and/or disorders.

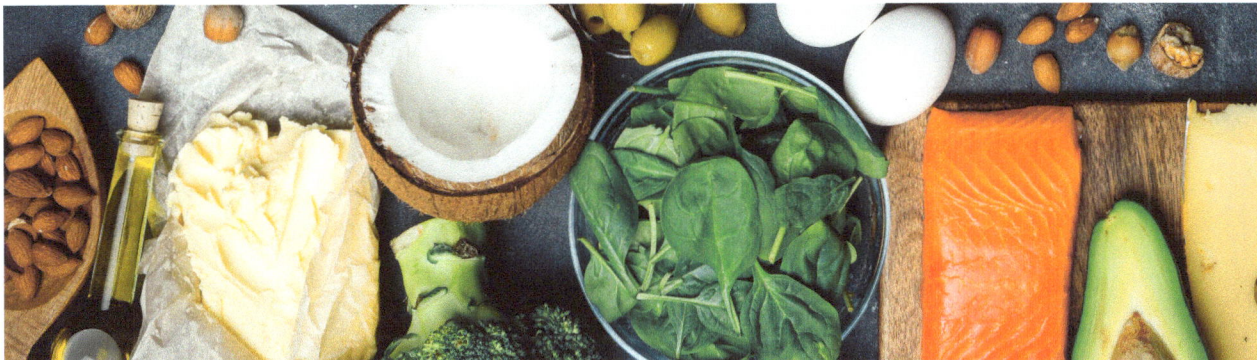

Micronutrients

Micronutrients are the vitamins and minerals your body needs to perform essential functions. Despite being required in relatively small amounts compared to macronutrients, micronutrients play a part in nearly every process in your body and are therefore essential for optimal health. They support several important functions, including growth, brain development, and immune functioning (preventing and fighting diseases).

Vitamins and minerals can act as antioxidants, which protect against cell damage associated with debilitating diseases including cancer, Alzheimer's and heart disease. Research has linked selenium deficiencies to a higher risk of heart disease, whereas multiple studies have shown that *adequate* calcium intake actually *decreases* the risk of death from heart disease and other causes.

For the most part, your body is unable to produce the essential vitamins and minerals you need, which means these substances must be obtained from your diet.

Since no single food source contains all the vitamins and minerals your body needs, it's important to eat a wide variety of foods to ensure you're getting the full range of micronutrients needed to support optimal health.

Types and functions of micronutrients

There are four types of micronutrients: water-soluble vitamins, fat-soluble vitamins, macrominerals, and trace minerals. All of them are absorbed into your body in similar ways and are involved in a multitude of bodily processes.

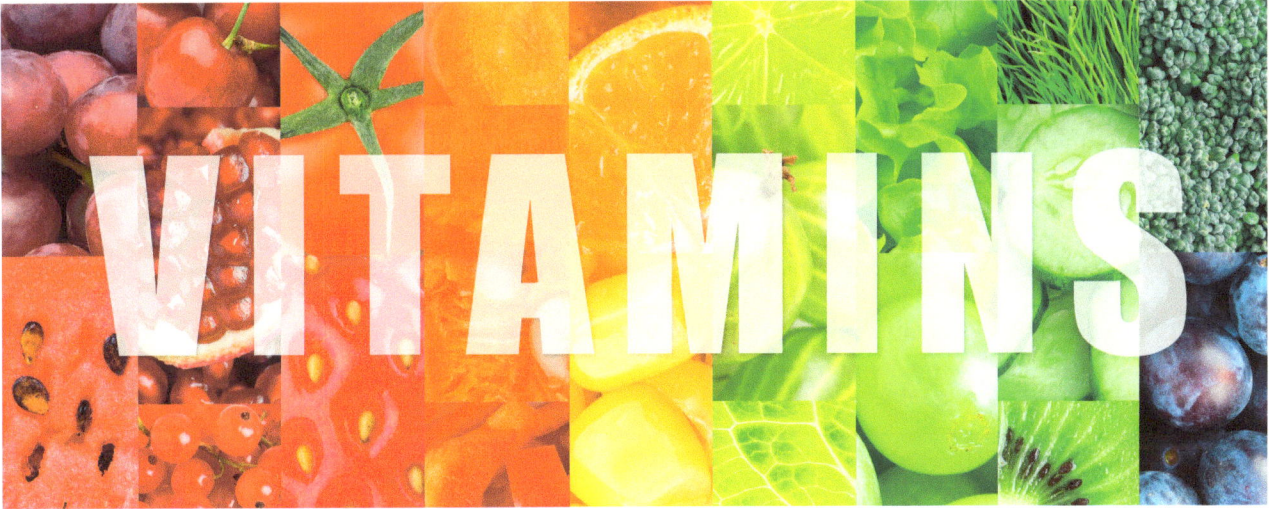

Vitamins and minerals

Vitamins are organic compounds made by the plants and animals we eat, whereas minerals are inorganic substances that are absorbed by plants and animals from the surrounding soil or water.

Vitamins

Vitamins play essential roles in helping your cells to convert food into energy. They also help to build proteins and promote cell division and tissue growth. They are used to produce collagen that keeps your skin healthy, heals wounds, supports blood vessel integrity, and promotes healthy bones and teeth.

Vitamins help your body to ward off and fight diseases. Without the required vitamins, your eyes, skin, lungs, digestive, immune and nervous systems cannot function properly.

Water-soluble vitamins

As the name implies, this category is made up of vitamins that dissolve in water, and it includes the majority of vitamins. They are required in large amounts from the diet as they cannot be stored in the body and are easily and frequently lost due to their water-soluble nature. When their concentrations in the body become too high, they are flushed out in the urine.

Water-soluble vitamins play important roles in energy production as well as other body processes, as shown in the table* below.

Water-soluble vitamin	Role	RDA/AI for adults over 19 years old	Good sources include
Vitamin B1 (thiamine)	Helps to convert nutrients into energy.	1.1–1.2 mg	Whole grains, meat, and fish.
Vitamin B2 (riboflavin)	Helps with energy production, cell function, and fat metabolism.	1.1–1.3 mg	Organ meats, eggs, and milk.
Vitamin B3 (niacin)	Helps convert food into energy.	14–16 mg	Whole meat, salmon, leafy greens, and beans.
Vitamin B5 (pantothenic acid)	Helps with fatty acid synthesis.	5 mg	Organ meats, mushrooms, tuna, and avocado.

Water-soluble vitamin	Role	RDA/AI for adults over 19 years old	Good sources include
Vitamin B6 (pyridoxine)	Helps with the production of red blood cells and facilitates energy production through the release of sugar stored in carbohydrates.	1.3 mg	Fish, milk, carrots, and potatoes.
Vitamin B7 (biotin)	Aids the metabolism of fatty acids, amino acids, and glucose.	30 µg	Eggs, almonds, spinach, and sweet potatoes.
Vitamin B9 (folate)	Assists with proper cell division.	400 µg	Beef liver, black-eyed peas, spinach, and asparagus.
Vitamin B12 (cobalamin)	Helps with red blood cell production, and proper nervous system and brain function.	2.4 µg	Clams, meat, and fish.
Vitamin C (ascorbic acid)	Helps with production of neurotransmitters and collagen.	75–90 mg	Citrus fruits, bell peppers, tomatoes, and Brussel sprouts.

Fat-soluble vitamins

These vitamins are stored in the liver and fatty tissues. They are insoluble in water and are best absorbed from the diet when consumed with fats and oils.

Roles, sources, and RDAs for fat-soluble vitamins are shown in the table* below.

Fat-soluble vitamin	Role	The RDA/AI for adults over 19 years old	Good sources include
Vitamin A	Helps with proper vision and organ functioning.	700–900 µg	Liver, dairy, fish, sweet potatoes, carrots, and spinach.
Vitamin D	Promotes proper immune functioning and helps with calcium absorption and bone growth.	15–20 µg	Sunlight, fish oil, and milk.
Vitamin E	Helps with immune functioning and acts as an antioxidant, protecting cells from damage.	15 mg	Sunflower seeds, wheatgerm, and almonds.
Vitamin K	Required for blood clotting and proper bone development.	90–120 µg	Leafy greens, soybeans, and pumpkin.

Minerals

Minerals help our bodies to maintain optimal fluid levels in tissues and cells. They also promote healthy bone formation and stabilise the protein structures that make up the hair, skin, and nails. Minerals move oxygen around the body and assist with the sense of taste and smell. There are two types of minerals: macrominerals and trace minerals.

Macrominerals

Macrominerals are needed in larger amounts than trace minerals.Roles, sources, and RDAs for macrominnerals are shown in the table* below.

Macromineral	Role	The RDA/AI for adults over 19 years old	Good sources include
Calcium	Essential for proper structure and functioning of bones and teeth. Assists with muscle functioning and blood vessel contraction.	2000–2500 mg	Whole dairy products, leafy greens, and broccoli.
Phosphorus	Building block for bone and cell membranes.	700 mg	Salmon, yoghurt, and turkey.
Magnesium	Assists with more than 300 different enzyme reactions, including regulation of blood pressure.	310–420 mg	Almonds, cashew nuts, and black beans.

Macromineral	Role	The RDA/AI for adults over 19 years old	Good sources include
Sodium	Helps maintain the fluid balance in cells and tissues and regulates blood pressure.	2300 mg	Table salt, processed foods, and canned soups.
Chloride	Used to make digestive juices, and, along with sodium, helps to maintain the balance of fluids in cells and tissues.	1800–2300 mg	Seaweed, table salt, and celery.
Potassium	Like sodium, it is an electrolyte that helps regulate the flow of fluids into and out of cells. It also helps with nerve transmission and muscle function.	4700 mg	Lentils, spinach, bananas, and avocados.
Sulphur	Found in every living tissue and is a key component of the amino acids, methionine and cysteine.	The RDA/AI not yet established.	Meat, poultry, fish, legumes, garlic, onions, eggs, and mineral water.

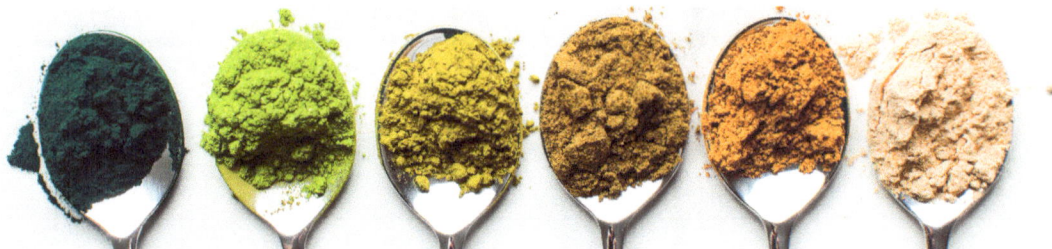

Trace Minerals

Although they are required in smaller amounts than macrominerals, trace minerals are vital for good health. Roles, sources, and RDAs for trace minerals are shown in the table* below.

Trace mineral	Role	The RDA/AI for adults over 19 years old	Good sources include
Iron	Assists in the transport of oxygen to muscle tissues and helps with the production of certain hormones.	8–18 mg	Oysters, spinach, white beans, and liver.
Manganese	Promotes the metabolism of carbohydrates, amino acids, and cholesterol.	1.8–2.3 mg	Pineapple, pecan nuts, and peanuts.
Copper	Used in connective tissue creation and plays an important role in normal brain and nervous system functioning.	900 µg	Liver, crab, and cashew nuts.

Trace mineral	Role	The RDA/AI for adults over 19 years old	Good sources include
Zinc	Promotes normal growth, immune function, and wound healing.	8–11 mg	Oysters, crab, and chickpeas.
Iodine	Essential to proper thyroid regulation.	150 µg	Seaweed, cod, and yoghurt.
Fluoride	Needed for the development of healthy bones and teeth.	3–4 mg	Fruit juices, crab, Australian tap water, and mineral water.
Selenium	Promotes thyroid functioning, reproductive health, and defence against oxidative damage.	55 µg	Brazil nuts, sardines, and ham.

*Source: Healthline, https://www.healthline.com/nutrition/micronutrients#types-and-functions, 2022

Micronutrient deficiencies

Despite only being required in tiny amounts, we don't always get all the micronutrients we need. Here, we'll take a look at some common micronutrient deficiencies.

Vitamin D deficiency

In a 2011–2012 health survey, the Australian Bureau of Statistics reported that one in four Australian adults suffered from vitamin D deficiency. The health effects of vitamin D deficiency include rickets in children and osteoporosis in adults. Low vitamin D levels have been linked to cardiovascular disease, chronic kidney disease, diabetes, multiple sclerosis, and certain cancers.

Age, skin colour, obesity, pregnancy, and low sun exposure are considered risk factors for developing vitamin D deficiency.

In most cases, vitamin D deficiency can be avoided by exposing areas of bare skin to sunlight. However, this is not recommended in countries like Australia, where the risks of developing skin cancer are high. In these countries, it's important to follow a diet rich in vitamin D and, when necessary, take oral supplements to prevent deficiencies.

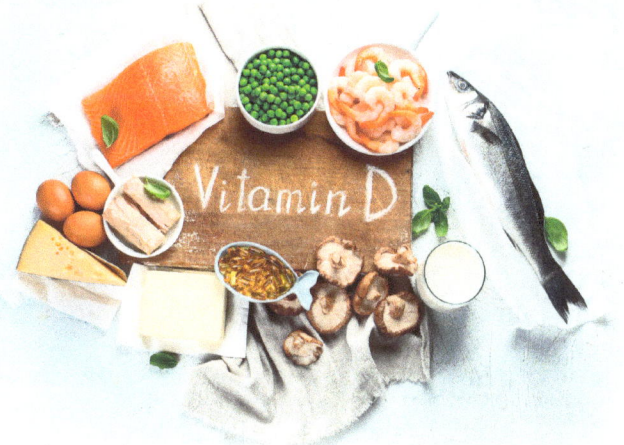

As there may be health risks associated with taking vitamin D supplements when they are not required, we strongly recommend consulting your healthcare practitioner to get this deficiency confirmed by blood tests before taking any supplements.

Iron deficiency

Iron deficiencies are common among children, pregnant and/or menstruating women, athletes, and vegans. Possible symptoms of iron deficiency include lethargy, fatigue, breathlessness, poor memory and concentration, susceptibility to infections, behaviour problems in children, and decreased libido in adults. Common causes of iron deficiency are blood loss, not eating enough iron-rich foods, and medical conditions, such as coeliac disease, that restrict the absorption of iron.

Your body needs iron to support a healthy immune system, mental function, muscle strength, and energy levels. Your body cannot produce its own iron, so it relies on your diet to provide the iron it requires. The best way to prevent iron deficiency is by eating iron-rich foods.

There are two forms of iron available from food: haem and non-haem. Haem iron comes from meat, poultry, and seafood. It is more easily absorbed by the body than non-haem iron, which is mainly derived from plants.

Haem iron can be supplemented by eating more red meats, organ meats, poultry, and eggs. Non-haem iron can be supplemented by eating more nuts, oats, tofu, dark leafy greens, dried fruit, and legumes (e.g., mixed beans, baked beans, lentils, and chickpeas). Combining iron-rich foods with those rich in vitamin C, such as citrus fruits, can aid in the absorption of iron from the diet.

We strongly recommend avoiding self-diagnosis when it comes to iron deficiency as taking iron supplements when they are not required can lead to health issues. If you suspect you may have iron deficiency, please consult your healthcare practitioner. They will be able to confirm your iron levels by means of a blood test.

Vitamin B12 deficiency

Vitamin B12 is not found in plants, which puts vegans (as well as some vegetarians) at risk of developing B12 deficiencies. People with medical conditions such as coeliac disease and Crohn's disease are also at risk as these conditions limit the absorption of vitamin B12 from the diet. Elderly individuals may also experience B12 deficiencies as their systems may not absorb this vitamin effectively.

Vitamin B12 is responsible for red blood cell production, normal nerve functioning, and DNA synthesis when cells divide. It is also important during pregnancy and breastfeeding.

A deficiency of vitamin B12 could lead to health complications, including anaemia (low red blood cell count), nerve damage, and neurological disorders. Symptoms of B12 deficiency include numbness or tingling in the hands, feet or legs, walking, lethargy, fatigue, light-headedness, pale jaundiced skin, and rapid heart rate.

The best sources of vitamin B12 are animal products, including red meat, poultry, seafood, eggs, and milk.

Plant-based foods fortified with B12 are available for vegans and vegetarians. These include soy milk products, yeast spread, yeast flakes, and vegetarian meat substitutes.

Please consult your general practitioner and get your vitamin B12 levels checked before taking any supplements.

Calcium deficiency

Over half of all Australians two years and older are not getting enough calcium, according to the *National Nutrition and Physical Activity Survey* of 2011–2012. It goes on to say that 73% of female Australians consume less calcium than is recommended compared with 51% of males.

Calcium takes up 2% of total body mass and plays a vital role in strengthening bones and teeth, regulating muscle and heart function (contraction and relaxation), blood clotting, the transmission of nervous system messages, and enzyme function. So, it's easy to see why maintaining optimal levels of calcium is so important.

Calcium deficiency weakens the bones, so they become brittle and more susceptible to breaks. Babies, young children, pre-teens, teenagers, and the elderly are at risk of calcium deficiency. Pregnant and breastfeeding women need calcium but do not normally need to supplement their dietary calcium since their bodies absorb calcium from food more effectively than other individuals.

Lifestyle risk factors for calcium deficiency include a high-salt diet, more than six caffeine containing drinks per day, excessive alcohol intake, very low body weight, very high fibre intake, low levels of physical activity, low levels of vitamin D due to lack of sunlight, and smoking.

Calcium is best obtained by eating a healthy balanced diet. Sources of dietary calcium include milk and dairy products, fortified milk substitutes, leafy green vegetables, soy and tofu, fish, nuts, seeds, and fortified breakfast cereals and breads. Calcium supplements at levels of 500 mg to 600 mg per day are both safe and effective at reducing the risk of fractures in people who don't get sufficient calcium from their diets. If you're concerned about calcium deficiency, consult your healthcare practitioner and have your calcium levels checked prior to taking any supplements.

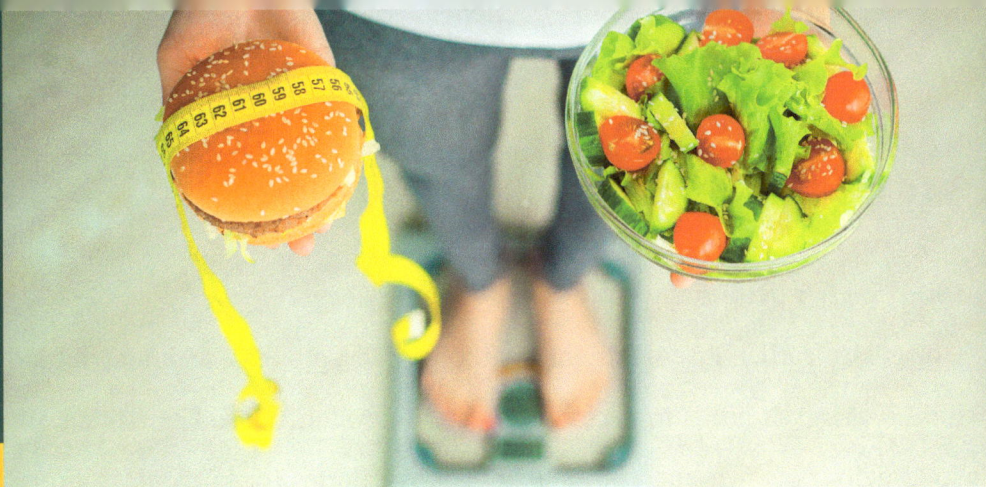

Eating for weight loss

What you put in your mouth, you wear as your body — so if you want a healthy body to rock a healthy life in, you better put healthy food in your mouth, period.
Michelle Bridges

The best and healthiest way to eat for weight loss involves covering your plate in colourful, delicious, healthy food. In this chapter, we'll share some pro tips to help you reach your goal weight and maintain your healthy body weight.

The journey to your healthy weight begins in the mind (but you knew we'd say that, didn't you?) Here are three quick mindset shifts that will help you to develop a healthy relationship with food, nurture a more positive body image, achieve your healthy body weight and maintain it long term.

Three mindset shifts for your weight loss journey:

1. Acknowledge and accept that lasting weight loss takes time.

2. Choose a balanced diet that fits your preferences, lifestyle, and goals.

3. Work patiently with your body to shed the extra kilos.

Eight steps to healthy weight loss

1. Make sure your body's getting the optimal amount of energy

As we discussed earlier, macronutrients (carbohydrates, proteins, and fats) in food provide your body with the energy it needs to perform its day-to-day functions. The amount of energy that each type of food delivers is measured in units known as calories (or kilojoules). Foods with high-calorie contents provide more energy to the body than those with lower-calorie contents.

Regularly and habitually consuming more calories than your body requires results in all those additional calories being converted into fat and deposited in fatty tissues under the skin, around vital organs (heart, kidneys, and liver), and along the walls of your veins and arteries. These fat deposits can lead to major health concerns and may ultimately be fatal.

In order to reach and maintain a healthy body weight and prevent chronic illness, you need to ensure that your body gets the optimal amount of energy from your food – no more and no less.

But, how do you know exactly how many calories you should be consuming each day?

There is no one-size-fits-all answer to this question. Everyone is different, and the exact recommended number of calories per day will depend on your age, activity level, and other metabolic factors. A qualified nutritionist or dietician will be able to assist you in creating the optimal meal plan to suit your unique requirements.

In general however, men need more calories than women, and active individuals need more calories than sedentary ones. Depending on their activity levels, healthy adult males of median height and weight with a BMI of 22.5 require between 2400 and 3200 calories per day. whereas healthy females of median height and weight, and BMI of 21.5 need between 2000 and 2400 calories per day.

2. Create a calorie deficit

In the simplest of terms, in order to lose weight, you need to set up a daily calorie deficit where "calories in" are less than "calories out". This means that the total number of calories you get from your diet (including all your food and drinks) must be lower than the total number of calories your body burns for that day.

Calories out include:

Calories burned at rest

This is known as your basal metabolic rate (BMR) and is calculated using standardised equations to determine how much energy your body uses at rest (i.e., when you're lying down, doing absolutely nothing). BMR calculations take your height, sex, age, and weight into account.

Calories burned during exercise

This includes "incidental" exercise, such as housework and walking around, as well as exercise that you do as part of your job, plus "intentional" exercise, such as jogging, aerobics, boot-camps, swimming, cycling, hiking or weight-training. Together, they make up your total daily energy expenditure (TDEE). This is calculated by multiplying your BMR by an activity factor determined by how active you are.

Calories in come from your diet

They are made up of all the calories in the food and drinks you consume. Food tracking apps make it easy to look up and track the number of calories in the food you're eating. Some apps even have a barcode scanning option that makes it incredibly easy to log your calorie intake for the day.

How can you lose weight sustainably?

In order to lose weight, it is important to ensure that the calories in your daily meal plan fall within the optimal caloric intake required to maintain your calorie deficit. That said, we don't advocate obsessive calorie counting or fad diets that involve extreme calorie deficits.

A healthy approach to creating a calorie deficit is to ensure that your calorie intake is 15% to 25% lower than your TDEE.

Remember to take your measurements before you start and at four-week intervals to monitor your progress. Keep a food diary and/or log your meals and exercise on an app to make sure you stay on track.

As a quick aside, if you're trying to gain weight, you need to create a calorie *surplus* by *increasing* your calorie intake so that it is 5% to 15% *greater* than your TDEE.

> " What comes easy won't last, and what lasts won't come easy.
>
> Unknown

3. Stay mindful of the fact that healthy weight loss takes time

It's normal to want to lose weight fast, but it's not sustainable. It took time to put the weight on, and the truth is, it's going to take a while to lose it in a healthy way. So, don't give up if you don't see results on the scales at every weigh-in. Keep going. You will get there.

Weight loss usually happens quickly in the first weeks of starting a weight loss program, and then it tapers off and may even plateau for a while before picking up again.

It's important not to lose heart and give up when things slow down on the scales. According to experts losing between 0.45 kg and 0.9 kg per week is a healthy and safe weight loss rate.

It may be frustrating, but, on the plus side, most experts agree that slow, steady weight loss is best when it comes to achieving lasting results. People who lose weight more slowly tend to keep it off in the long term. And slower weight loss carries fewer health risks.

4. Exercise cannot compensate for overeating or following an unhealthy diet

If you aimed to lose one kilogram over a week by focusing on exercise alone, without paying attention to your diet, you would need to burn a minimum of 7700 calories. To do that, the average adult would need to run at 10 km/hr for about 15.2 hours or do 17.5 spin classes each week. When you think about it that way, it's easy to see that trying to burn off 7700 calories through exercise alone is not going to work. Relying solely on your training program to create such a huge calorie deficit would be near impossible. Exercise alone won't get you the weight loss results you crave. You need to follow a healthy diet too.

You cannot out-run a bad diet.

Michelle Bridges

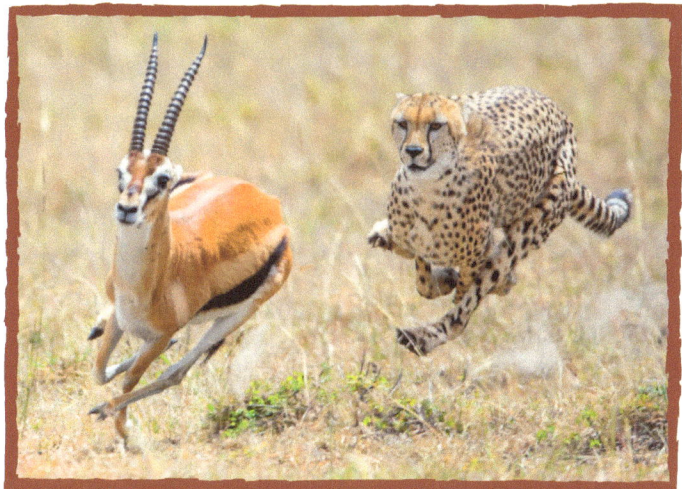

5. Starving your body will not speed up the process

> **" Ye cannae change the laws of physics.**
> **Chief Engineer Scotty from Star Trek**

Exercise alone won't accelerate weight loss and neither will starving yourself, depriving yourself of certain foods, or even eating only one type of food.

Take Dave for example. As a fairly active average adult male, Dave burns roughly 2000 Cal per day. If he were to try to lose one kilogram of fat in a week, he would need to create a calorie deficit of around 1100 Cal per day for seven days. To create this 1100 Cal deficit solely by dieting, Dave would only be able to consume 900 Cal (in both food and drink) per day for the whole week. That would mean virtually starving himself. While it is entirely possible to do this, it's not at all healthy or sustainable.

Losing weight too fast through extreme calorie deficits like this will only lead to a host of poor outcomes, including muscle loss, sluggish metabolism, fatigue, weak and brittle bones, hair loss, gallstones, brain fog, lowered immune response, illness, and chronic health issues.

Yo-yoing between weight loss and weight gain is another common side effect of extreme calorie-deficit diets. After a few days or a week on one of these super restrictive diets, you're likely to over-eat and put all the weight you just lost back on again – and then some. Plus, if your diet makes you feel weak and sickly, you're not going to stick to it. And...

The number one reason why most diets fail is that people are unable to stick to them long-term.

6. Limit your intake of "empty" calories and macros

Scientifically, one calorie is very much like another, but from your body's point of view, the source of your daily calories is very important. The same goes for macros. Just because no foods are off-limits, doesn't mean that all foods are equal.

When choosing between 100 g of buffalo wings (yum) and 100 g of salmon (also yum), there's not much difference when you only consider the macros. Both dishes contain 60% protein and 40% fat, but when you look at the bigger nutritional picture, it's easy to see that you're not going to get all the essential nutrients you need if you choose the buffalo wings every time.

That's because food does more than just fuel the body with energy (calories), it also provides vital minerals and nutrients that the body needs to function properly and ward off infection. Sweet potatoes and lollies both consist of 100% carbohydrates. Pick the lollies over the sweet potato, and you may be hitting your macro target for carbs, but you're not getting the fibre, vitamins, and minerals found in the sweet potato.

The highly refined and processed foods (e.g., cakes, cookies, lollies, donuts, processed meats, energy drinks, soft drinks, ice cream, sweetened fruit drinks, fast foods, crisps, and chips) that flood the market today may taste good and provide more than enough calories (and macros) to keep you going, but they lack the crucial nutrients that you need to survive.

> **"** You are what you eat, so don't be fast, cheap, easy or fake.
>
> Unknown

Consumed in excess, these foods represent significant health risks and have been shown to increase the incidence of heart disease, cancer, and chronic illness.

The calories from these foods are essentially "empty" calories as they have little to no nutritional value. To reduce the number of empty calories you consume, try to limit foods that contain mainly refined sugars, saturated fats, trans fats, refined grains, and high levels of sodium.

Added sugars and saturated fats should each comprise less than 10% of your daily calorie intake and sodium levels should be kept below 2300 mg per day.

Now, remember when we said there are no good or bad foods? Well, we're not contradicting that statement here. You see, it's not the type of food that's the problem – it's the ingredients. Pizza, for example, can be made from highly processed nutrient-poor ingredients, slathered in fatty oils, and covered in sugary sauces – an empty calorie meal if ever there was one. But a homemade pizza, from fresh organic ingredients, such as spinach, kale, sweet potato, mushrooms, and capsicum, topped with low-fat cheese on a cauliflower base delivers a nutrient-dense food that is healthy and enjoyable.

7. Choose nutrient-dense foods

This step is really the magic sauce when it comes to reaching and maintaining a healthy body weight. We have already covered this in great detail in the chapter on balancing your diet, so we'll just remind you here that when looking for nutrient-dense foods, you should seek out real, unprocessed, whole organic foods that are not manmade, have not been chemically altered, and do not contain any synthetic ingredients. These foods should form the bulk of your diet.

8. Reduce or remove alcohol from your diet

When it comes to weight loss, alcohol is not your friend. In fact, it is quite often responsible for weight gain because it's easy to forget to include calories from alcohol in our daily calorie intake tally. And, when it comes to empty calories, alcohol packs quite a punch (pun intended): a whopping seven calories per gram, which is almost as much as a gram of pure fat. Plus, when you add in the calories from sugary mixers (e.g., cola, lemonade, orange juice or tonic water), suddenly your knock-off drinks are taking a chunk out of your daily calorie for very little nutritional reward.

To make matters worse, it's hard to keep track of the number of drinks you're consuming, especially when you're at a party or in a big group. Plus, it's a fact of life that one ever goes out for a salad after a big night. You're far more likely to stop by the local kebab shop or dial your favourite fast food delivery service and order up the giant pizza with extra cheese or a massive burger with extra fries, plus an ice cream sundae and a milkshake, or anything big, cheesy, greasy, and calorific.

Fortunately, there is an excellent array of non-alcoholic drinks to choose from. These range from simple but refreshing low-calorie soda and fresh lime to more exotic and complex mocktails. Choose from old favourites such as a "Virgin Bloody Mary" or "Virgin Mojito" or try your hand at creating your own signature drinks. Just go easy on the sugar syrup.

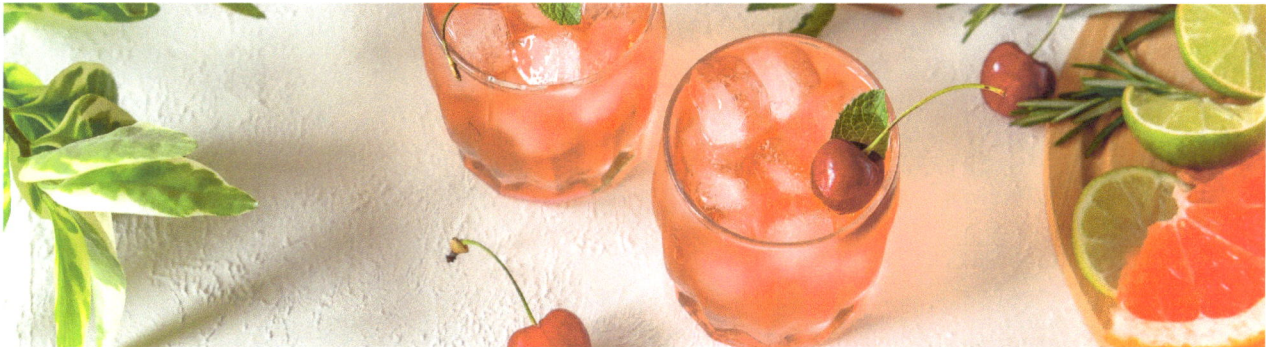

Alcohol guidelines

According to the Australian Alcohol and Drug Foundation, there is strong and consistent evidence that alcohol causes cancers of the breast, liver, colon, rectum oropharynx, larynx, and oesophagus. Even low levels of drinking can increase your risk. That does not mean that drinking alcohol will definitely give you cancer, but it *does* increase your risk. Reducing your alcohol intake or not drinking at all can significantly lower your risk and help you live a healthier life.

Guidelines developed by the National Health and Medical Research Council (NHMRC) recommend that, in order to reduce the risk of harm from alcohol-related disease or injury, Australians should:

- Drink no more than 10 standard drinks per week.

- Consume no more than four standard drinks in a single session.

- Anyone under 18 should not drink alcohol to reduce the risk of harm to the developing brain.

- Women who are pregnant or breastfeeding should avoid alcohol to prevent harm to their babies.

What constitutes a standard drink?

A standard drink consists of 12.5 ml of pure alcohol, which equates to:

- Spirits 40% alcohol, 30 ml nip

- Wine or sparkling wine 13% alcohol, 100 ml average serving

- Full strength beer 4.9% alcohol, 285 ml glass

- Light beer 2.7% alcohol, 425 ml glass

- Cider 4.9% alcohol, 285 ml glass.

How to lose weight by tracking and calculating your macros

Macronutrients include proteins, carbohydrates, and fats in various forms, which release energy when digested by the body. Many people these days prefer to track and calculate their daily intake of macronutrients, instead of counting calories.

When using macronutrient tracking to lose weight, you need to determine the appropriate ratio of macronutrients based on your current body weight and required calories.

The *2015–2020 Dietary Guidelines for Americans* recommend the following ratios for the average adult:

- Carbohydrates: 45% to 65% of calories
- Fat: 25% to 35% of calories
- Protein: 10% to 30% of calories

However, there is no one-size-fits-all magic macro ratio that guarantees weight loss for everyone. Your individual ideal protein-fat-carb ratios will depend on a host of different factors, including your age, sex, activity levels, state of health, and weight loss goals.

One popular way of tweaking your macros for weight loss involves adjusting the carbohydrate-to-protein ratio so that it prompts your body to reduce fat deposits and add lean muscle tissue. This works because, calorie for calorie, protein offers the biggest metabolic hit for weight loss by increasing the feeling of satiety, preserving muscle mass, and stimulating energy expenditure (i.e., helping the body burn more calories).

While your body absolutely *does* need carbs and fats to power your cells through the day (particularly when you're working out), by reducing your carbohydrate and/or fat intake and increasing the amount of lean protein you consume (within reason), you'll be encouraging your body to build lean muscle mass and reduce body fat.

The recommended daily allowance (RDA) of carbohydrates is 130 g per day. This represents the minimum amount of carbs required to fuel the average adult brain, red blood cells, and nervous system. This means you need at least 130 g of carbs each day for your body to function normally. Don't be tempted to dip below the RDA because, if you reduce your carbohydrate intake too much, your body will fuel your brain and red blood cells by converting proteins into glucose.

Certain types of excess protein may be stored as fat, which can lead to weight gain. Plus, many high-protein foods are also high in saturated fat and total fats, which can result in elevated blood lipid levels and heart disease.

Also, beware of pumping protein levels up by too much because an excess of protein in your diet will be broken down into amino acids that are excreted in urine. This puts strain on your kidneys.

Dieticians recommend scaling the ratio of carbs to proteins down from 50:20 to 45:25 Let's take a look at an example to show how this works.

Sarah is 40 years old, moderately active, and wants to lose weight. Based on her BMR and TDEE, she needs 1200 Cal from her diet each day to promote healthy weight loss. If Sarah reduces the percentage of calories from carbs in her diet from 50% to 45%, and ups her protein intake from 20% to 25%, she will still be consuming 135 g of carbohydrates each day, which meets the RDA of 130 g for adult women.

Any further reduction in her carbohydrate intake will put her below the RDA, making it difficult to hit her daily fibre goal. This will lead to lethargy and fatigue – especially during workouts.

Once you know how many grams of each macro you should consume every day, it's easy to track your food and ensure that you're hitting your daily targets. We'll take a closer look at exactly how to track your food and drinks in the next chapter. In the meantime, let's talk about cravings.

What can you do to overcome food cravings?

We've all been there. It's four o'clock in the afternoon, and you're hard at work, minding your own business, when suddenly you're overcome with a craving for [*insert your favourite treat here*]. It could be a delicious donut, a chocolate chip cookie, a slice of pie or cake, an apple fold-over, a packet of crisps or a slab of chocolate. What do you do? You want to stay focused and stick to your diet, but the feeling just won't go away. Here are a few strategies you can use to overcome food cravings and give yourself the best chance to succeed in your weight loss goals.

1. Know your triggers and plan ahead

Cravings often rock up after a particular trigger has occurred. For example, in the afternoon when energy levels dwindle *or* at times of high stress *or* when a bus goes by with an ad for a new variety of chocolate *or* you walk past several vending machines every day and, every time you do, those packets of crisps, chocolate bars, and cookies cry out to you.

Spend a week tracking your eating habits, including when you ate, what triggered you, what you ate, and why. Don't try to change anything while doing this exercise, just note your cues and triggers. Once you have identified them, you can plan your meals and snacks ahead of time and adjust your daily habits, so you can avoid these cues and triggers and stay on track with your nutrition.

2. Have healthy snacks on hand

Cravings are also creatures of habit, rolling around at more or less the same time every day. If you know you're going to crave a snack at a particular time of day, make sure you've packed a delicious and healthy alternative in your lunch box. Have it ready to whip out and enjoy when the craving hits.

The best way to prepare for this is to set some time aside on the weekend to create a meal plan for the week. Include three meals and two snacks for each day. Purchase only the foods you need to fill your meal plan. Pack your food up into servings ahead of time, so you can easily grab what you need for the day each morning before you head out the door.

3. Shop the perimeter of the supermarket

Most supermarkets have a similar layout with fresh produce, dairy, meat, and fish sections on the perimeter of the store and processed foods in the centre aisles. An easy way to reduce your intake of empty calories is to shop exclusively on the outskirts of the store, focusing on fresh, whole, healthy produce and avoiding the inner aisles where processed foods lurk.

Unpackaged foods such as fresh meat, fish, poultry, fruit, and vegetables should fill up the bulk of your trolley. Be selective about foods that come in packaging. Choose those with four or fewer ingredients on the label, and avoid those with unpronounceable ingredients.

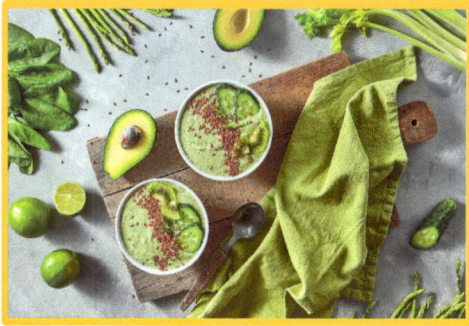

Meal Planner

	BREAKFAST	LUNCH	DINNER	SNACKS	DRINKS
MON					
TUE					
WED					
THU					
FRI					

4. Choose fruit and/or vegetables over sugary snacks

Fruit and veggies travel well, are nutrient dense, and make great alternatives to lollies or chocolates when it comes to satisfying cravings for sugary foods at work or school.

By offering up fresh fruit, veggies, whole grains, and lean proteins to your tastebuds every time you crave a snack, your palate will gradually become accustomed to these foods. Over time, they will feature more prominently in your cravings, taking the place of the empty calorie foods that you used to crave. Keep at it and, within a few weeks, the highly processed foods will no longer interest you.

5. Fill up on healthy fats

If that apple in your desk drawer just doesn't cut the mustard when it comes to satisfying your cravings, consider making your afternoon snack time the time when you treat your body to some healthy fats. Try a handful of trail mix, mixed nuts, almonds or cashews. Alternatively, snack on an avo, some fresh guacamole or a can of fatty fish, such as salmon or tuna. Healthy fats will fill you up and keep you full much longer while reducing your cravings.

Craving something salty? Popcorn (air-popped, not microwave), roasted edamame or fava beans or wholegrain crisp breads with cottage cheese tomato or cucumber and salt all make healthy low-calorie alternatives to potato or corn crisps that are often high in saturated fats.

6. Pack protein into your diet

Another way to overcome cravings is to fill up on proteins instead of reaching for carbs. Grab some fish, beans, lentils, chickpeas or nuts when you're hungry, and you'll feel satisfied for longer.

7. Interrogate your cravings

When you feel cravings coming on, it's important to interrogate where they come from.

Remember the two types of hunger we discussed before? Are you experiencing hedonic hunger or true hunger? In other words, do you feel like eating because your body needs food or because you're stressed out, depressed, bored or overwhelmed?

Has this craving been triggered by an advertisement you saw for junk food, a vending machine filled with empty calories in alluring wrappers, or some other cue or trigger?

By probing your feelings of hunger and questioning your cravings for certain types of food, you're exercising your mindfulness muscles and healing your relationship with food.

When you start making more informed choices about whether or not you're going to eat and what foods you're going to put into your mouth, you'll feel a renewed sense of self-worth and self-confidence, knowing you can trust yourself to make the right choices for your body.

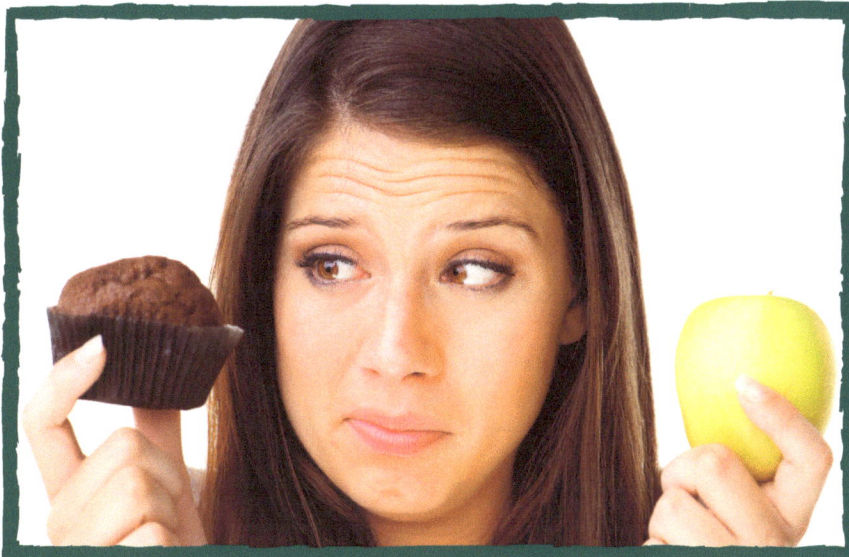

8. Introduce new coping strategies

Use these strategies to banish hedonic hunger and cravings:

- Switch out unhealthy snacks for healthy ones.

- Take some deep breaths or do a short meditation.

- Go for a walk to clear your head.

- Take a break and do something creative, such as sketching or colouring in.

- Get some exercise or do yoga.

- Talk to a friend or colleague about what's bothering you.

- Ask for help when struggling with an issue or dealing with an overwhelming workload.

- Tell yourself that you can have that snack later on (chances are the craving will pass, and you'll forget all about it).

- Wherever possible, find and take new routes that reduce your exposure to advertising triggers or vending machines. Even better if these new routes add to your step count. And while we're on the subject of advertising, try to avoid the ads on prime time commercial "free-to-air" TV. They're invariably trying to convince you to buy fast foods filled with nothing but empty calories.

9. Focus on what you *can* have rather than what you're trying to avoid

Studies indicate that it is easier to overcome cravings by crowding out thoughts about the foods you're trying to remove from your diet with thoughts about the foods you want to include.

When a craving hits, try to think about all the foods you *can* eat, instead of thinking about the foods you're trying to reduce. It's likely you'll find something healthy to satisfy your craving this way.

10. Get more sleep

Lack of sleep often drives your cravings for refined and processed foods. The body signals that it's tired and needs more energy, and the brain urges you to get that energy in the fastest way possible – through easily digestible sugary or fatty foods.

By getting more sleep, you can actually reduce these cravings. If you are sleepy and craving sugars or fatty foods, remember that reaching for refined foods will do more harm than good. They will only pick you up for a brief moment before allowing you to go crashing back down into exhaustion again. Try to satisfy those cravings for energy with slow-burning nutrient-dense foods instead, and you'll not only feel better, but you will also have more energy for longer.

11. Spice things up

Another way to reduce food cravings is to keep adding new and varied foods to your diet. Trying new dishes, experimenting with different spices and flavours, and keeping things interesting will prevent boredom and reduce cravings for refined and processed foods. Eating a wide variety of foods (include different colours and textures) will improve your overall health and boost immunity.

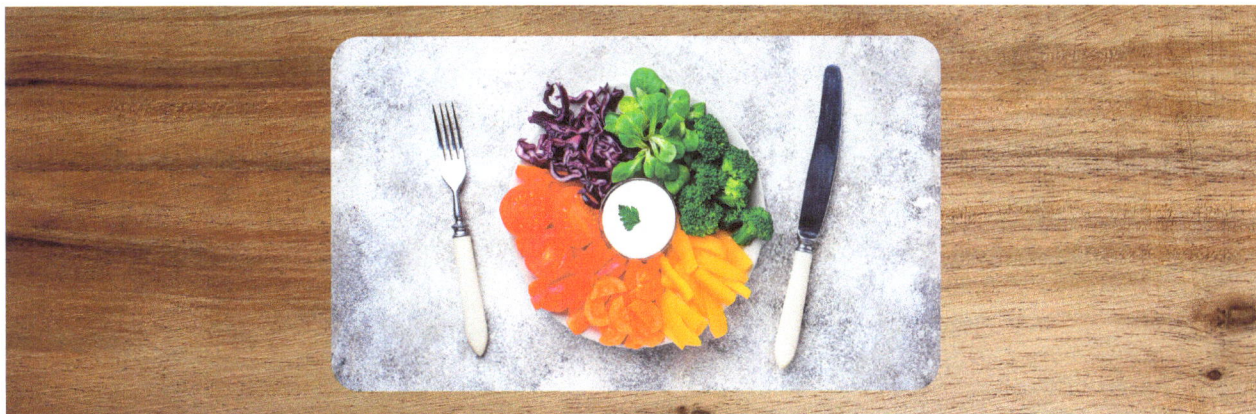

12. Stay hydrated

Your body is designed to require food once every three to four hours. If you're hungry more frequently than that, you could be dehydrated.

It's common to experience hunger pangs, when, in fact, you are dehydrated. The confusion between the two sensations happens in a part of the brain known as the hypothalamus. It is responsible for detecting and interpreting the body's signals for hunger and thirst. When the hypothalamus gets its wires crossed, you may end up feeling hungry when you're actually thirsty.

The easiest way to discover whether you're truly hungry or thirsty is to make drinking a glass of water your default response to hunger pangs. If you feel satisfied after drinking water, you were probably just thirsty. If not, reach for a healthy snack to tide you over until mealtime. Not a fan of plain water? Try drinking it with a twist of lime or lemon, add a few mint leaves, or make an infusion of green, herbal or fruit teas.

If neither the water nor the snack satisfies you, you're likely experiencing hedonic hunger, and it's time to question why you feel compelled to eat. Are you bored? Depressed? Anxious? Triggered? Try going for a walk, chatting to a friend or colleague, or doing some breathing exercises or yoga to help you relax. Or try one of the other coping mechanisms mentioned above.

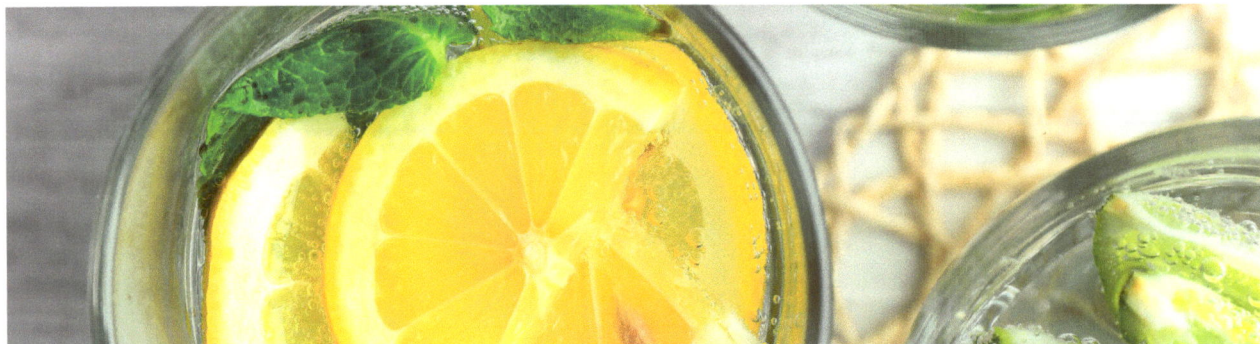

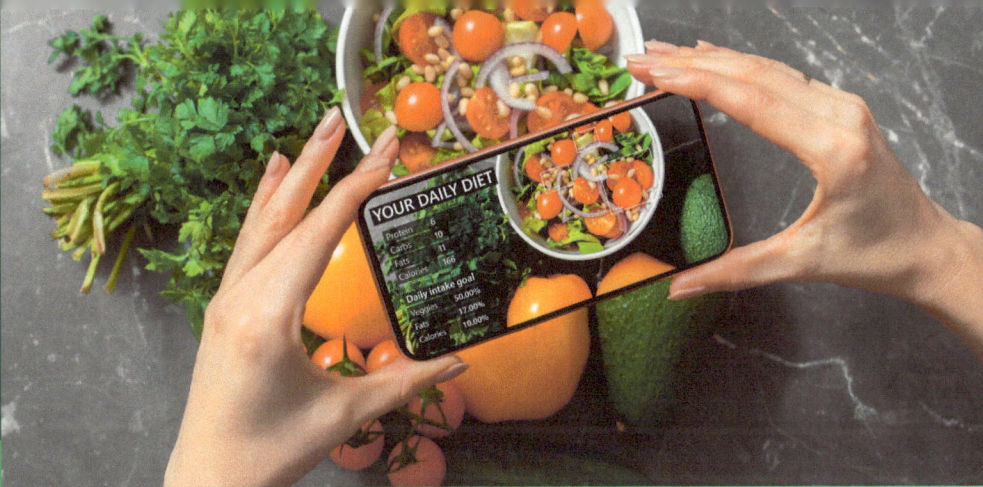

Food tracking

If it goes in your smacker, put it in your tracker.
Unknown

Food tracking gives you the knowledge you need to start your healthy eating journey from a position of power, fully aware of your current food habits. Try it for one day or even a week without making any changes to your diet. Don't judge or try to eat a certain way, just observe.

Track everything you put into your mouth – food and drink. You'll soon discover the quality of your foods, and whether you've been consuming more (or fewer) calories than you thought.

Once you've established a baseline, try keeping a daily food diary as you work on improving your relationship with food. This habit provides a simple but effective way to ensure your body's getting the right nutrients, and your calorie and macro intakes remain within the healthy range.

Benefits of food tracking

1. A clear picture of your eating habits

Food tracking is the key to understanding your eating habits, discovering where the issues lie, and finding ways to fix them. Knowing where you are right now – what your food triggers are, the nutrient composition of your food, and how many calories, macro- and micronutrients you're consuming – will help you discover what needs to change to improve your overall health.

2. Weight loss

Daily food tracking may hold the key to achieving your weight loss goals. According to research conducted by a popular fitness tracking company, 88% of people who tracked their food for a week on their food-tracking app lost weight, and those who tracked more often, lost more weight.

Here's why: It's easy to consume additional calories every day without even thinking about it. You probably know that eating a double cheeseburger, fries, and a milkshake for lunch will blow out your daily calorie allocations, but did you know that a large hazelnut latte with no sugar, contains more calories than a 46 g chocolate wafer bar? (250 Cal vs 230 Cal)

Add sugar and cream to your latte, and you're looking at an extra 500 calories a day – just from your morning coffee. That's 3500 Cal every week, which is equivalent to almost half a kilogram of fat – every week.

When you're not mindfully tracking your food, you'll happily grab a coffee each morning on the way to work without paying much attention to all those extra calories.

So, if you think you're eating healthily, but you're still not losing weight, be on the lookout for hidden calories. They could be the reason you're getting nowhere fast.

Hidden calories often come from drinks – a latte here, a soft drink there, an energy drink before work, or a beer or wine in the evening. But they can also be found hiding out in the foods that we mindlessly snack on.

Who doesn't love tucking into a couple of bikkies at morning tea, a handful of charity chocolates in the afternoon, or a bag of crisps while watching TV? Without tracking, sneaky snacks slip in under the radar and stop us from achieving our weight loss goals.

Even foods that sound healthy, like a grilled chicken and salad wrap, can come with a hefty calorie count (in some cases up to 1000 Cal) that takes a huge bite out of your daily allowance.

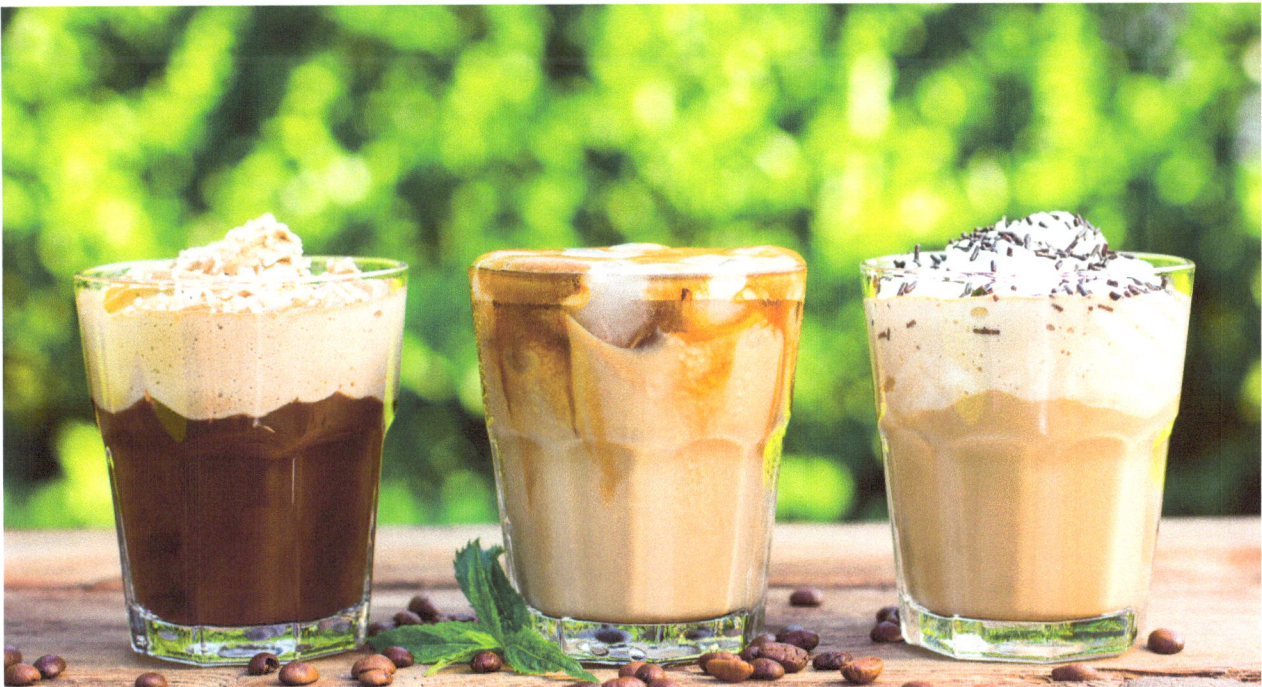

3. More mindful eating

Can you remember what you had for dinner last night? How many beers you had at the party on the weekend? Or, for that matter, all the things you snacked on during your busy day at work today? How often do you find yourself eating on autopilot as you hurry through your day – too busy to pay attention to what you're putting in your mouth?

Tracking your food intake helps you to be more mindful of your eating and drinking habits. Knowing that you will be recording what you eat and drink, makes it easy to intervene when you're about to reach for a high-calorie drink or nutrient-poor snack out of habit or boredom.

4. Really get to know your food

When you use a food tracking app, you get inside information about each item of food or drink you're consuming – not just the calories, but also the macro- and micronutrient content. This helps you make more informed choices about what to include in your diet and what to leave out.

It won't take long before you start seeing those dreamy donuts for the big fat sugar bombs that they truly are, rather than the glossy delicacies you once believed them to be. When you really get to know your food, it's easy to make better food choices and create a new way of life.

5. Stay hydrated

Are you drinking enough water? After tracking your water intake for a couple of days, you may be surprised to find that you're not really drinking as much as you thought. Tracking will help you to optimise your water intake and stay hydrated.

6. Be empowered to make healthy food choices

Once you get the hang of your chosen food tracking app, you'll be able to use it to plan your meals ahead of time, make informed choices, and work the foods you love into your daily and weekly menus in optimal amounts. Your body will reward you by functioning better than ever.

7. Reveal any food intolerances

By tracking your meals and noting how you feel after each meal, you'll be able to identify the foods that leave you feeling bloated, experiencing stomach pains, constipation, diarrhoea, IBS, eczema or other symptoms. Once you're aware of your particular food intolerances, you can create a healthy diet that excludes foods that make you feel unwell.

8. Identify triggers that lead to overeating

Do you always pour yourself a beer or a glass of wine when you get home? Do you raid the fridge when everyone else has gone to bed? Do you reach for a chocolate bar when you're stressed or bored at work? By tracking your food intake, you'll begin to notice the triggers, such as stress, habit or boredom, that lead you to overindulge or binge.

These food triggers are easily identified as they are not related to real hunger or thirst, but to cravings, habits, and emotions. Food tracking can help you to see them for what they really are. Once identified, you can use your coping strategies to overcome them. For example, a good way to conquer hedonic hunger and cravings is to engage in activities that don't involve eating or drinking, such as playing sports, spending time with your family, listening to music, watching TV or reading.

9. Recognise the links between eating habits, cravings, and fatigue

Do you struggle to keep your eyes open in the afternoon? Or battle food cravings in the evening? Perhaps you hit the wall mid-morning and inevitably reach for a chocolate bar or croissant to pick you up? These things may not seem to be related to your eating habits, but after tracking your food and drink intake for a while, connections may emerge.

For example, the mid-morning slump is often a result of not eating a nutritious breakfast. Carb-loading at lunchtime could cause you to feel drained in the afternoon. And skipping supper could be the cause of late-night bingeing. Whatever your situation, tracking your food will help reveal the ways you can tweak your diet and your habits, so you feel energised each day and sleep well at night.

10. Measure your progress

Best of all, food tracking allows you to see your progress. Not only in terms of making healthier food choices and reaching a healthy weight but also in terms of your energy levels, sleep health, and hydration levels.

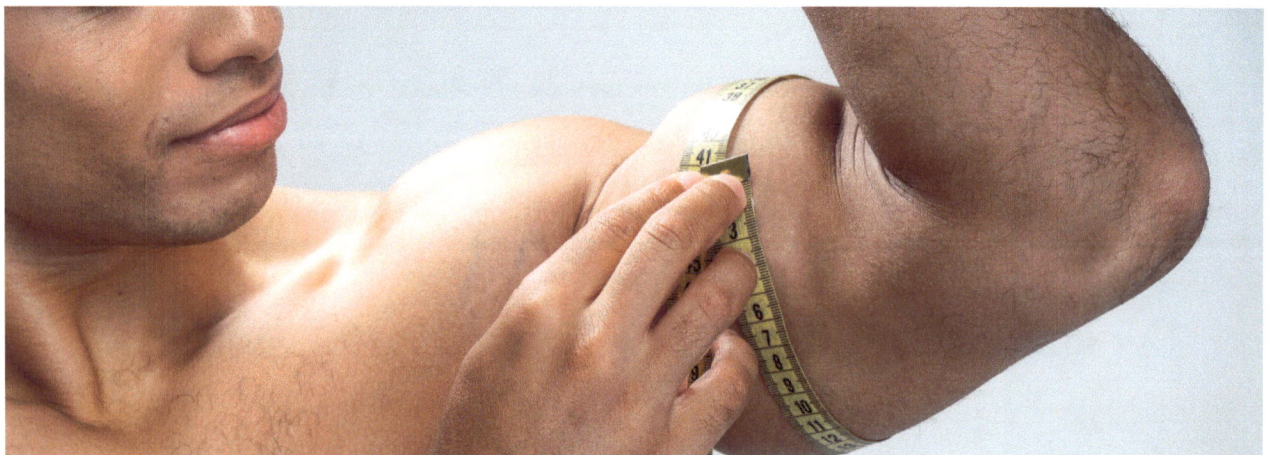

How to track your food and drinks

1. Find a food-tracking app or process that works for you

We've mentioned (more than once) the benefits of having an app to track your nutrition. That's because they're so easy to use. Nutrition apps provide access to extensive food databases and include other useful features such as barcode scanners that make it easy to log the foods you eat. The easier it is to track food and drinks, the more likely you will be to keep on tracking.

There are plenty of apps out there, including some that cater to specific nutrition choices, such as vegan or keto.

Search your app provider and try out a few different apps until you find one that meets your needs.

The great thing about having an app on your phone is that you always have your phone with you, so there's no excuse *not* to track foods while you're out.

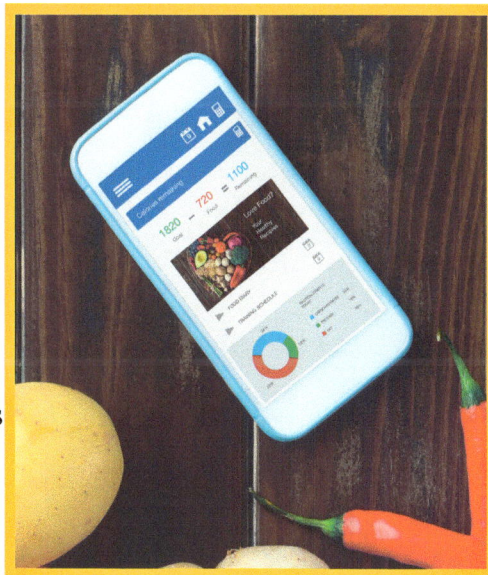

Not a technophile? No worries. Grab a diary or notebook and a pen or pencil and track your food intake manually. You can look up the calorie content, macros, and micros using the search function on your web browser or refer to the Nutritional Information on the package.

2. Set up a baseline

Start by simply tracking without trying to make any changes to your diet. After a week, you'll have a baseline. Then make small changes, one at a time, and see how they add up to great results.

3. Track often

The more you track, the better your results will be. So, make a habit of tracking each meal, drink or snack as soon as you have it. That way you won't miss anything. It might seem to be a bit of a hassle at first but be patient. Keep at it until it's second nature.

4. Don't get bogged down in the details – just keep tracking

A reliable food tracking app should have an extensive database of foods that you can use to find and track your food and drinks. But don't get too bogged down with trying to find the exact food item you have on your plate. It's completely okay to choose something that's similar to what you're eating. Tracking something is better than tracking nothing at all, so go for it.

5. Don't beat yourself up – just keep tracking

So, you had a two pieces of pie at Sally's baby shower. No need to panic, just track it and move on. You may have to reduce your calorie intake for the remainder of the day – no big deal.

You can even use your trusty food tracking app to look up some of your favourite foods and see what types of foods and portion sizes will fit into your remaining calorie allowance for the day. Then it's just a simple matter of following your revised eating plan for the day.

6. Use your tracker to craft kick-ass meal plans

You can use the app to create delicious and nutritious meal plans that will fuel your body for the day and keep you feeling healthy, happy, and satisfied, while still enjoying the foods you love.

7. Set mealtime reminders

If you struggle to take time out of your schedule for meals, set mealtime reminders, either through your food tracking app or using the reminder function on your phone or computer. This is a great way to ensure that you're nourishing and hydrating your body regularly throughout the day.

8. Celebrate your successes (and keep tracking)

If you've achieved a positive change in your eating habits, celebrate. Whether it's a great result at your weekly weigh-in, finally closing the top button on your favourite pair of jeans or not polishing off the leftover birthday cake in the fridge, take a moment to acknowledge your victory.

Taking time out to reflect on how far you've come will help keep you motivated and encourage you to make more healthy choices in future.

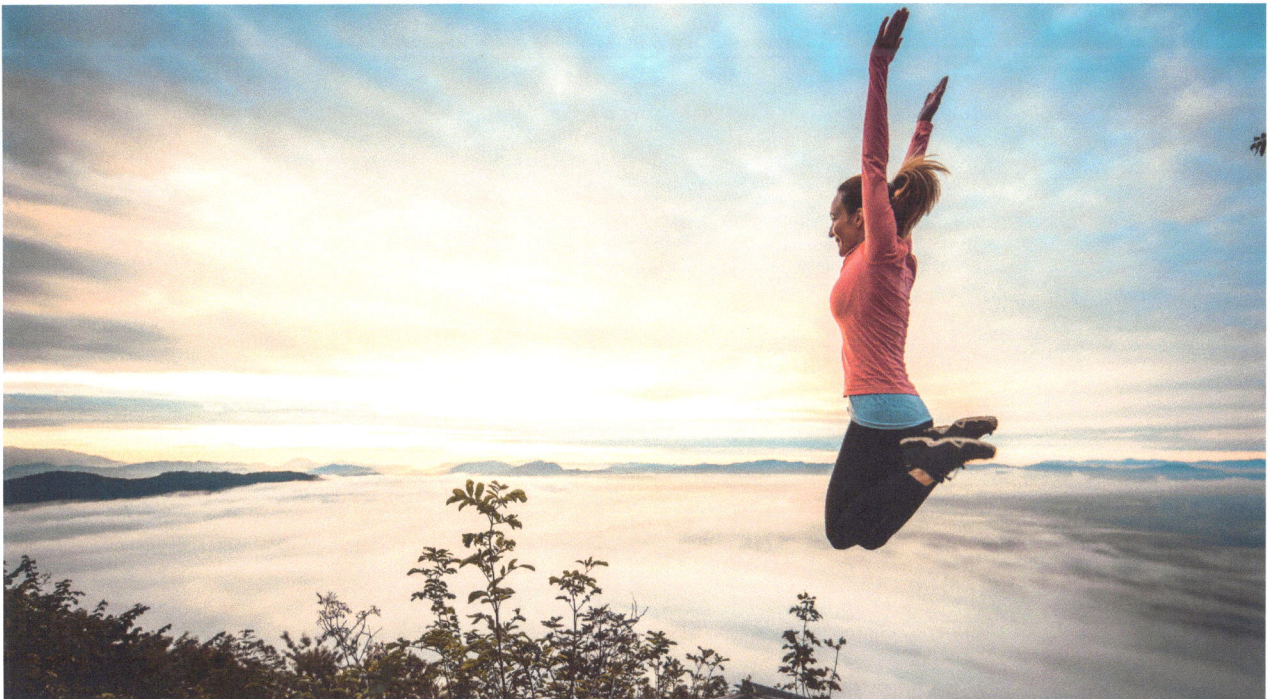

NOTES

Believe. Train. Nourish. Achieve.

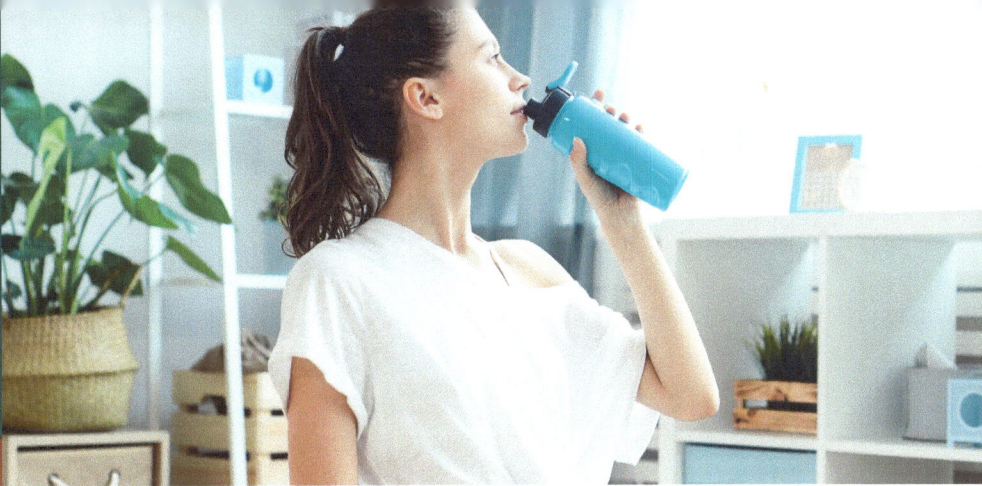

Hydration

In one drop of water are found all the secrets of all the oceans.

Khalil Gibran

The importance of hydration

1. Water is the elixir of life

Water makes up about 60% (by weight) of the human body, and it is essential for the proper functioning of all internal systems. While you can get by for weeks without food, dehydration can kill within days or even hours.

2. Water promotes healthy bodily functions

It helps your liver and kidneys to get rid of toxins, regulates body temperature, keeps joints lubricated, and helps to prevent infections.

3. Water keeps your cells healthy and functioning

Water flows into and out of cells during normal bodily functioning, delivering vital nutrients and removing waste products and toxins.

4. Your body is constantly losing water

Water leaves the body via breathing, sweating, urination, and bowel movements. Along with water, you are also constantly losing sodium, magnesium, potassium, and other salts. Known as electrolytes, these substances are vital to proper cell functioning.

5. Dehydration affects your ability to function

When more water leaves the cells than enters them, you become dehydrated. Mild dehydration can occur after just 30 minutes of exercise and affect your body's ability to function properly. As dehydration progresses, it may lead to fatigue, brain fog, constipation, kidney stones, and urinary tract infections.

6. Hydration promotes weight loss

Drinking water regularly throughout the day helps your brain to accurately identify thirst and send the correct signals, so you don't feel hungry when you're actually thirsty.

Water contains zero calories per gram, making it ideal for settling hunger pangs without taking a chunk out of your daily calorie budget.

A glass of water before each meal helps to fill up your stomach, making it easier to eat smaller portions. This lowers your calorie intake and promotes weight loss.

7. Dehydration triggers headaches and migraines

Studies indicate that lack of water in your body can trigger migraine episodes. Also, headaches last longer when your body is low on fluids.

8. Dehydration affects the brain

Dehydration affects brain functioning and can lead to brain fog, inability to concentrate, and trouble with short-term memory.

9. Dehydration affects mood

Dehydration affects mental health and can leave you feeling anxious, moody, and depressed.

10. Dehydration affects sleep

When you're well-hydrated, your sleep quality is better. Staying hydrated will help to ensure that you're getting more rest, feel more energised and are better able to cope with your days.

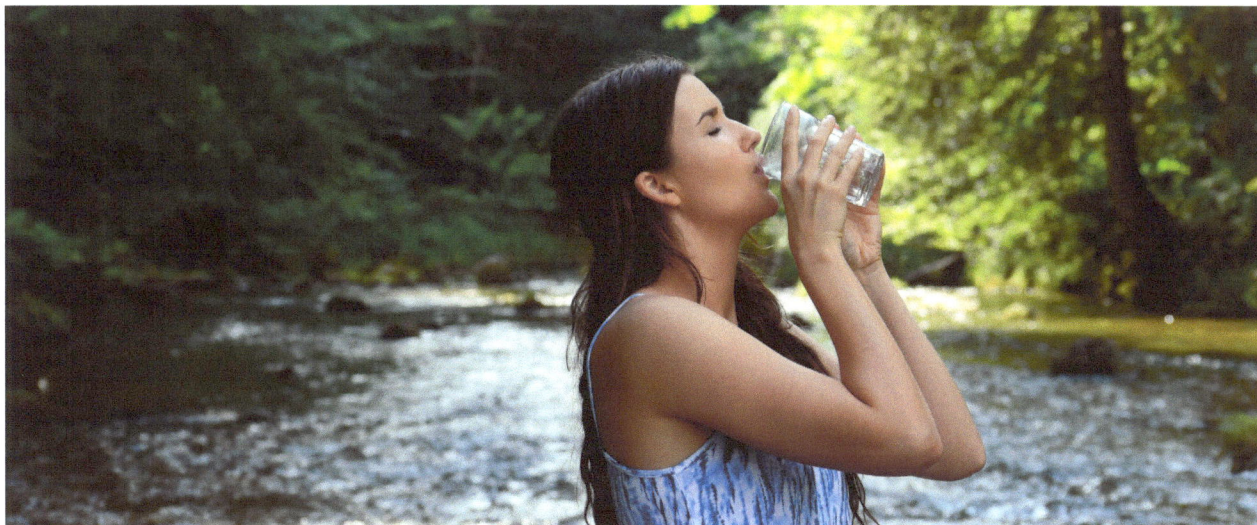

Dehydration – know the signs

1. Infants and young children

It can be difficult to recognise early signs of dehydration in infants and young children. In addition to providing regular hydration, loved ones and carers should be on the lookout for the following signs: irritability or lethargy, the absence of tears when crying, no wet nappies in the past three hours, dry mouth and tongue, sunken eyes and cheeks, and shrinking of the soft spot at the top of the infant's head.

2. Adults

Feelings of thirst are the obvious first signs of dehydration in adults. However, it's important to note that by the time you feel thirsty, your body is already dehydrated. Hunger, especially directly after completing a meal, is often a sign that you are dehydrated.

Other signs of dehydration include less-frequent urination, dark-coloured urine, headaches, fatigue, dizziness, confusion, and dry lips, mouth, and tongue.

Urine colour and dehydration

One way to ensure your body is properly hydrated each day is to check your urine colour. Morning is the best time to get a good indication of your hydration status using the colour of your urine. Healthy urine from a well-hydrated person will be clear and pale yellow in colour.

3. The elderly

Older adults may not feel thirsty, even when they are dehydrated. Carers should keep an eye on elderly people to ensure that they remain properly hydrated.

Hydration – it's not all just about water

Remember the days when you were told to drink eight glasses of water per day? Well, these days experts recommend 2.7 litres of fluids per day (women) and 3.7 litres of fluids per day (men).

Sounds a lot, doesn't it? But on the plus side, these estimates cover a wide variety of sources including plain water, tea and coffee, soups, other beverages, and also some of the water-rich foods you eat (e.g., watermelon, cucumbers, iceberg lettuce, celery, and tomatoes).

Watch out for carbonated soft drinks, sports drinks, energy drinks, vitamin waters and fruit juices though. One of the worst things you can do when dehydrated is to try to make up for drinking water by drinking loads of these. Even though some of them sound like healthy options, these drinks do more harm than good because of their high sugar content. In high doses, they are liable to wreck your metabolism, causing chronic conditions (e.g., diabetes). Caffeinated and alcoholic drinks have diuretic properties and are therefore also no good for hydration.

Let's look at some of the fluids you can drink to keep your body hydrated and healthy.

So, what's the best way to stay hydrated?

A healthy daily fluid plan should primarily consist of water. However, there is room for a few other fluid sources – ideally in the following ratios.

1. Water – plain and simple (>50%)

Of the roughly three litres of fluids required daily by the adult human body, experts recommend that at least half of that (1.5 litres) should be pure water – there's your six to eight glasses a day right there. Still as true as ever.

While drinking plain water is without a doubt the best way to stay hydrated – it's readily available and has zero calories – it's not always the most fun.

Some people will happily sip away at their water bottles, day in and day out, while others are repelled by the thought of drinking "plain old, boring old" water all day long. According to the experts, you can blame societal conditioning for driving your tastebuds away from the enjoyment of nature's own life-giver. Apparently, we don't like the taste of plain water simply because it doesn't deliver the desired hit of sweetness we've come to expect from our drinks.

If you're not a fan of plain water, try sprucing the flavour up by adding fresh berries, mint, lemon, cucumber or lime.

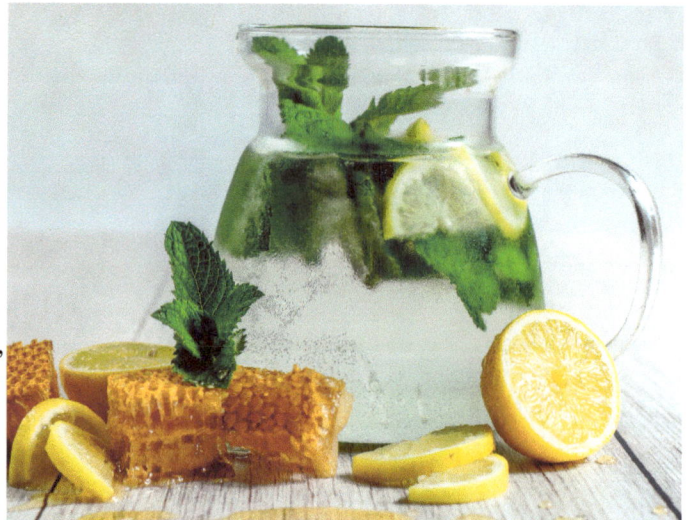

Ways to top up your water intake

- To keep costs down and save the environment from plastic water bottle waste, carry a reusable bottle of water around with you during the day or have one on your desk. Top it up with fresh water from a water filter or use tap water.

- Add some natural flavourings to your water by infusing it with fresh berries, slices of lemon or lime, crushed mint leaves or cucumber slices.

- Stack your water drinking habit with other daily tasks to make it easier to remember to drink water throughout the day. For example, drink a glass of water first thing in the morning, one at lunch time, and another with dinner. Drink one more just before bed. And make sure you drink water before, during, and after your workouts.

- Drink water when you feel hungry. This will help you to discern whether your hunger is real or whether you're actually thirsty. Real hunger will not be satisfied by drinking water. And, even if it is true hunger, the water you drink will help you feel full quicker making it easier to eat less and consume fewer calories.

- Set reminders on your phone or computer or invest in a drinking bottle that has time markers and/or motivational quotes on it to keep you topping up.

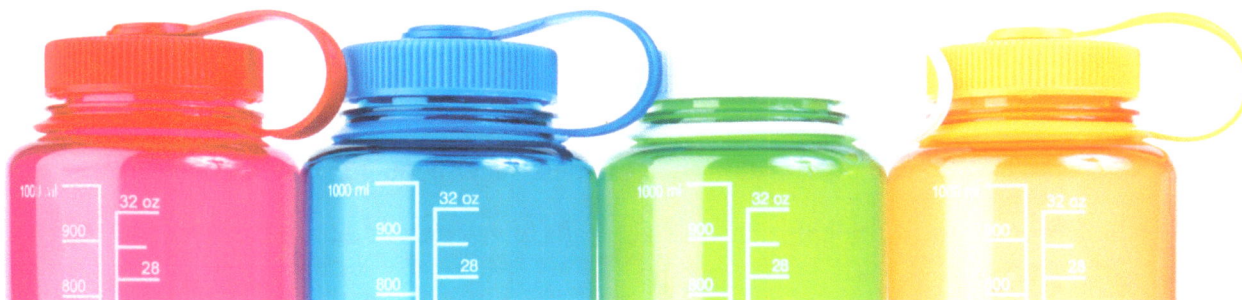

2. Unsweetened herbal infusions, tea or coffee (25%)

The good news (for some) is that approximately 800 ml of the remaining 1.5 litres of daily fluids can come from herbal infusions, tea or coffee – provided you skip the cream and sugar.

Go easy on caffeinated beverages. The caffeine and tannins in tea and coffee act as diuretics meaning that they increase the frequency of urination, which contributes to dehydration. Plus, drinking loads of caffeine throughout the day could leave you jittery, struggling to concentrate, and unable to sleep at night. So, try to limit the number of coffees per day and stick to low-caffeine or caffeine-free options, such as herbal or green teas.

3. Milk and/or milk substitutes (20%)

Your daily fluid intake can include up to 500 ml of low fat, skim, rice, almond or soy milk. This covers the use of these products in smoothies, tea and coffee, or over healthy cereals such as oats or muesli.

4. Fresh, natural fruit and veggie juices (5%)

The remainder of your intake can be made up of fruit or vegetable juices and/or the occasional artificially sweetened drink. Choose fruit and veggie juices that are freshly squeezed and as close as possible to their natural state since these have higher nutrient levels and no added sugar.

Avoid alcohol, sugary, carbonated or high-fructose drinks

Notably, the daily fluid plan contains no alcoholic, sugar-containing or high-fructose drinks as these provide no nutritional value, contain loads of calories, and are harmful to the body.

Hydration tips for active people

Active people need to pay particular attention to their hydration levels as exercise raises body temperature and increases water loss through sweating.

Water helps to transport nutrients to cells, enabling them to keep energy levels up while you work out. It also lubricates the joints and regulates body temperature to prevent overheating. Without proper hydration, your body will struggle to perform at its peak.

Dehydration has a marked effect on mental and physical performance:

- Dehydration causes your heart rate and body temperature to increase.

- Exercise seems to require greater exertion (particularly in hot conditions).

- Your form suffers and mental fatigue increases, which impacts decision-making and coordination of movement. This could lead to injury when performing exercises that require skill.

- As dehydration progresses, the risk of nausea, vomiting, diarrhoea, and other gastrointestinal issues also increases.

Hyponatraemia

Hyponatraemia is a rare, but life-threatening condition that occurs when athletes (usually those taking part in long-duration sports, such as ultra-marathons or long-distance swimming events) drink too much water and fail to replace the electrolytes lost during exercise. The overabundance of water in the body dilutes the concentration of sodium in the blood. This impairs cellular functioning, leading to headaches, disorientation, nausea, inability to urinate, and ultimately, coma and death.

How much water is required before, during, and after exercise?

It is important to create and maintain optimal hydration and electrolyte levels in your body before, during, and after exercise. You need to consume enough water and electrolytes to compensate for those lost during exercise.

Several factors play a role in how much you need to drink when exercising, including individual sweat rates, intensity levels, duration of exercise, heat, and humidity of the environment.

Basic hydration guidelines

To work out the exact fluids you need to perform at your peak, it's best to consult an accredited sports dietician.

These recommendations by the American Council on Exercise serve as a guide:

1. Drink 500 ml to 600 ml of water two to three hours before you start exercising.
2. Drink one glass of water 20 to 30 minutes before you start exercising or during your warm-up.
3. Drink another glass of water every 10 to 20 minutes during exercise.
4. Drink a large glass of water no more than 30 minutes after you exercise.

Approach sports drinks with caution

In most cases, plain water is sufficient to keep you hydrated during exercise. However, those involved in endurance sports, such as long-distance running or swimming or cross-country skiing, may need to top up their electrolytes during long intense training sessions to prevent hypernatraemia.

As a rule of thumb, if you're training at high intensity for more than an hour, you should supplement your water intake with an electrolyte drink. These may be purchased from sports nutrition stores in powder or tablet form and made up with water to the prescribed concentration.

Choose drinks have the relevant electrolytes in the right concentrations without too much added sugar and preferably without caffeine. Reach out to your nutritionist for advice on the best choice of electrolyte drink to suit your specific requirements.

Be sure to choose wisely when purchasing per-mixed commercial "sports drinks" such as those found at your local servo or convenience store. Not all drinks that are marketed as sports drinks are truly healthy. Bear in mind that so-called "energy drinks" are not suitable for use as electrolyte drinks. They often contain large amounts of sugar and caffeine as well as other ingredients (guarana, ginseng, taurine) that overstimulate the body and are not recommended as part of a healthy diet.

Pay close attention to the nutritional information on the container to ensure that you are actually getting the required electrolytes. Also, be aware of serving sizes. A single can or bottle could contain multiple servings, which means you will need to multiply the number of calories by the number of serves per bottle to get a true value of what you'll be consuming if you're going to drink the whole thing.

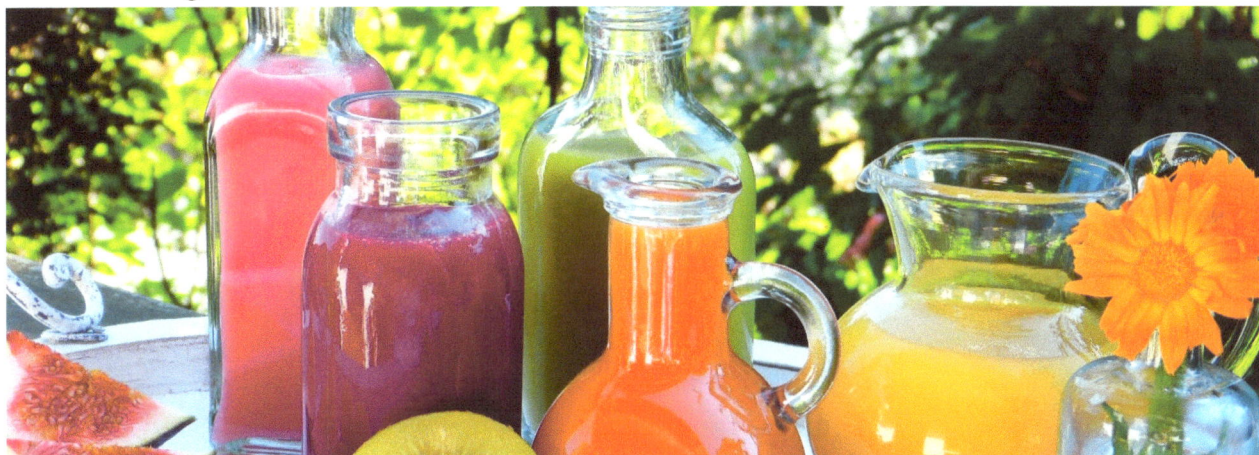

NOTES

Believe. Train. Nourish. Achieve.

Achieve

Review your
progress

Reward your
successes

Renew your
goals

Conclusion

NEW GOAL

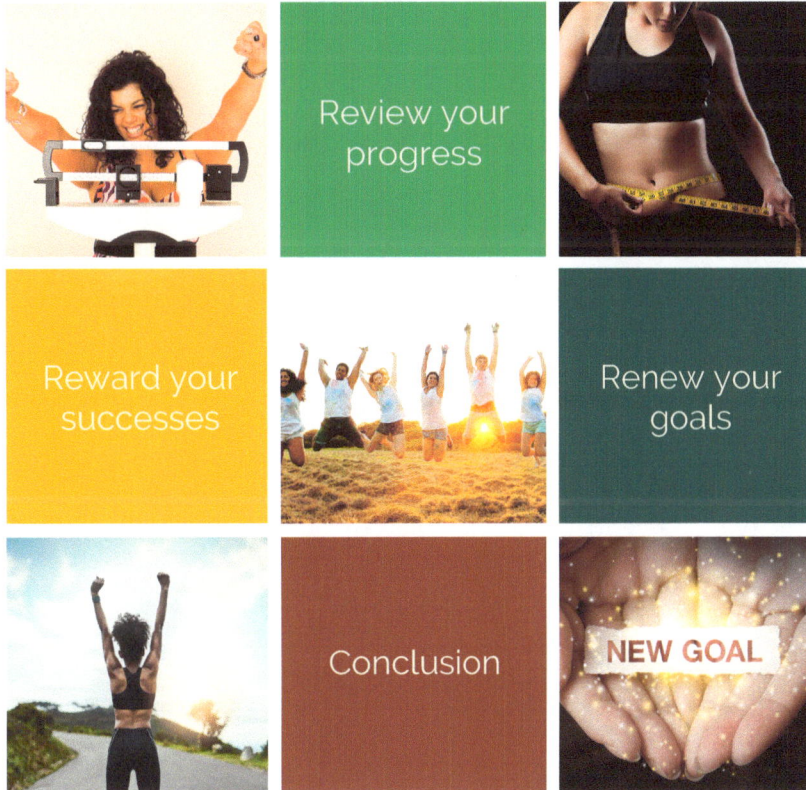

66 Remember to celebrate milestones as you
prepare for the road ahead.

Nelson Mandela

In this final section, we're going to explore the processes of assessing your progress, reviewing your results, and celebrating your successes – both big and small. Finally, we'll take a look at how to revise, refresh, and renew your goals, so you're constantly growing and evolving into the best possible version of you.

Remember those goals we set back in the Believe and Train sections of this book? Well, it's time to haul them out, along with your vision boards, goal statements, affirmations, wellness assessments, measurements, photos, tracking apps, journals, and everything else you've used to plan, track, and monitor your progress. Once you have gathered it all together, you're all set to discover how to use these tools to measure, evaluate, and celebrate your achievements. And, you'll be ready to set new goals and plan for an even brighter future.

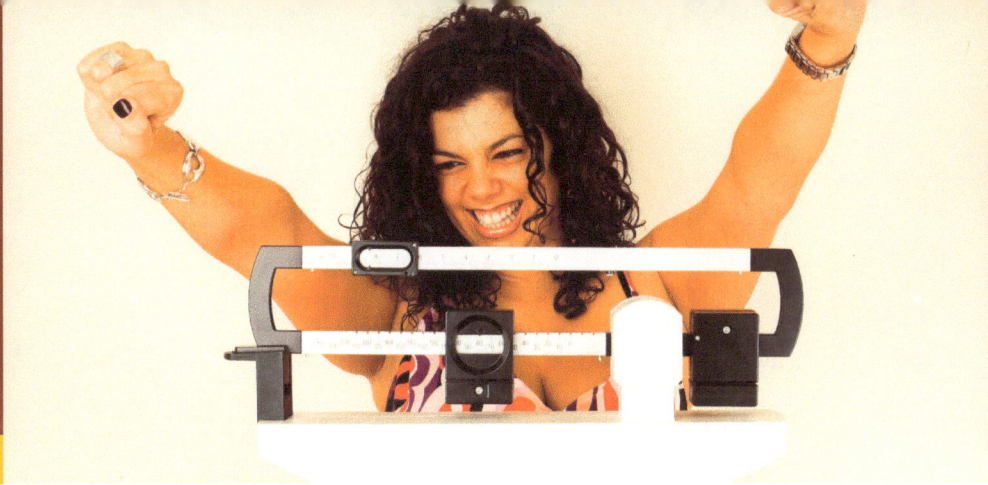

Review your progress

It's one thing to set a goal. It's another, however, when you get so caught up
in the details that you neglect to review your progress.
Re-evaluation enables you to improve your aim to ensure you hit your target.
Susan C. Young

No matter whether you're just a couple of weeks into your new health and fitness program or you've been chasing down a specific goal for years, it pays to take some time out every now and then to reflect on and review your progress.

In this chapter, we're going to take you through the benefits of regular progress reviews. We'll share some positive ways to tap into the power of the review process, and we'll show you how you can use that power to create the life you've always wanted.

Benefits of regularly tracking and reviewing your progress

1. Tracking your metrics and reviewing your progress reminds you of your goals

We all know just how easy it is to make goals AND how quickly and easily those same goals, no matter how well-intentioned, can be forgotten or procrastinated.

Regularly tracking and reviewing your progress helps to remind you of your goals and why they are important to you (*your why*).

For example, keeping a food journal, tracking your measurements, and/or having a target item of clothing that you want to fit into by a certain date will remind you of your weight loss goals.

Similarly, saying your affirmations out loud each day and regularly examining your vision board will remind you of the reasons you wanted to lose weight in the first place. These daily habits will help you find the strength you need to resist that triple cheese burger and loaded fries.

Another great way to track your progress is to use a novel visual aid. For example, you could decorate a jam jar with stickers and bling, then place one marble in the jar for every kilogram you want to lose. Remove a marble each time you lose a kilo. Keep the jar somewhere you can see it as a reminder of how you're tracking.

Reviewing your progress at regular intervals (e.g., weekly, monthly and annually) will keep your goals top of mind during the tough times when your initial enthusiasm has subsided.

> **"** To set goals is human, to stick to them is divine.
>
> Adapted from Alexander Pope's famous quote

2. Reviewing your progress motivates you to keep going

Success is a powerful motivator that fuels your desire to keep going and do even better.

W*ithout* regularly monitoring and reviewing your progress, you will *never* know what you've achieved so far, and whether you'd had any small successes that should be celebrated. You'll be denying yourself the motivational boost that comes from acknowledging and celebrating the small, incremental improvements that add up to bigger successes. If you're only focussed on your big goal, ignoring small wins along the way, you run the risk of becoming disheartened and feeling as though you're not making any progress.

3. Reviewing your progress helps you to learn from your failures

It's important to go through the process of reviewing your progress – regardless of whether it's been a good week or not – simply because you learn more from your failures than from your successes.

Facing up to your failures can be a challenge, especially if you demand high levels of performance from yourself and your body. But, by interrogating your failures, you'll be able to find out what led to them in the first place, and unearth the lessons contained in them. Sure, success motivates us, but failure shows us where there's room for improvement, and that's gold.

Our greatest glory is not in never falling, but in rising every time we fall.

Confucius

4. Reviewing your progress reveals stumbling blocks – and how to remedy them

Regularly reviewing your progress gives you the opportunity to identify and address any obstacles or challenges you've faced and see how they've affected you in terms of achieving your goals. This is especially useful after periods when you've failed to stick to your goals, skipped training sessions or when life has just managed to get in the way. Reviewing will help you to find ways to overcome the challenges, work around the obstacles, and avoid the pitfalls next time around.

5. Reviewing your progress helps you to overcome fears and overwhelm

Chasing down big goals takes courage, patience, and time, and it's possible to feel overwhelmed and afraid that you may never get there. Imposter syndrome, fear, doubts, and stress can gang up on you and try to beat you into submission. Regularly checking in with yourself, reviewing your progress, and mapping out the next steps on your journey can have an amazingly calming effect, allowing you to recharge and refocus.

In this way, reviewing reduces overwhelm and makes it easier to cope with the demands of chasing those big goals while juggling life at the same time. It also helps to put things into perspective, alleviates any fears and doubts around whether or not you're capable of achieving your goals and helps you to find the courage you need to keep going.

6. Reviewing your progress helps you to change course when necessary

A progress review can also show you when you've been heading down the wrong path and need to change direction. For example, imagine that you've been trying to lose weight through a rigorous exercise routine. After four weeks, you conduct a progress review, only to discover that you haven't reached the goal weight you set for the four-week mark, and you have sustained several injuries along the way.

A thorough review of your metrics and the challenges, obstacles, and setbacks you faced will help you get to the bottom of what is really going on. Perhaps you've been trying to out-train a bad diet. Or you've been overeating in an attempt to prop up failing energy levels that have arisen due to all the exercise you're doing. Reviewing your diet and exercise program will help you to make the necessary changes and get back on track. This could also be a good time to check in with your life coach, personal trainer and/or nutritionist for professional advice on how to tweak your programs to optimise your results.

> **"** If someone is going in the wrong direction, he does not need motivation. He needs to stop.
>
> Leonard Lebere
> (Adapted from Jim Rohn)

7. Reviewing your progress encourages you to ask questions, investigate, and find answers

Once you've examined your results and the entries in your various journals, you'll have a clear picture of what you've achieved, overcome and/or fallen victim to during the review period. This will coax you to ask and answer the pointy questions about your performance, your commitment, and your willingness to make changes. For example, have you been choosing nutrient-dense foods over empty calories? Are hidden calories in your food or drinks sabotaging your weight loss goals? Have you *really* been too busy to follow your program this week? Or have you been waiting for motivation? It will also reveal the things you need to do to improve your future outcomes.

8. Reviewing your progress helps you to map out the next steps

Once you know how far you've come, where you've fallen short of the mark, and the things that have caused you to stumble, you will have all the information you need to clearly map out the next steps in the journey towards your big scary goals.

Questions to ask in your review that will help you to see where you could tweak things to improve your outcomes include:

- Are there regular excuses that keep coming up and prevent you from doing the daily things that will get you closer to your goals?

- How can you reframe these excuses and/or work around them and start smashing your goals?

- What steps should you take to avoid the stumbling blocks, such as late afternoon chocolate binges at the office, that keep tripping you up?

- What events are coming up (e.g., periods of solo parenting, the festive season, Easter, annual holidays, birthdays, family functions, work functions, project deadlines, busy periods at work, kids' activities) that you need to be mindful of? What plans can you put in place to stay on track during these periods? Are there support systems you can call on? Can you delegate certain tasks? Can you put some less important activities (e.g., time spent watching TV or playing games on your phone) on hold so you've got time to focus on your goals while attending to these things? What self care measures can you put in place to ensure you can cope mentally and physically?

9. Reviewing your progress helps you to keep aiming higher

Regularly reviewing your progress not only keeps you accountable, it also helps you to keep setting new goals, raise the bar a little higher, and continue creating your best life.

How to track and review your progress

1. Track everything that relates to your goals and milestones

The success or failure of your mission to achieve your personal, professional, financial, health, fitness and any other big scary goals hinges on how well you track.

Unsure about what you should be tracking? Use the mini-goals and milestones set up in the Goal Setting chapter of this book (pp 51–76) to establish your metrics.

> **Quick tip** Don't hit the scales too often. Weight fluctuates quite a bit from day to day. Stick to weekly weigh-ins for the best measure of your progress.

Tracking your metrics is just the beginning though. To get a clear picture of your progress, you need to track the context in which that progress has (or has not) taken place. In other words, in addition to tracking the food you eat, the exercises you're doing, the number of glasses of water you drink, the number of times you've trained or practiced, you also need to track the challenges and obstacles you've faced, your moods, your workloads, and your attitudes. Heck, you can even track your kids' moods and your pets' attitudes. In short, track *everything* that has an effect (whether positive or negative) on achieving your goals.

> " If you cannot measure it, you cannot improve it.
>
> Lord Kelvin (aka William Thomson)

There are plenty of ways to track your progress. Here are a few examples:

- **Apps:** Take your pick of hundreds of virtual apps that make tracking easy.

- **Pen and paper:** Treat yourself to a brand-new journal and get tracking.

- **Measurements:** For weight loss, track your weight, waist, chest, arm and thigh measurements.

- **Photos:** Take photos of yourself at the start and at regular intervals throughout your program.

- **Target outfit:** Select an item from your wardrobe that you would like to slim down into. Try on your target outfit and take photos at regular intervals to show your progress.

- **Visual aids:** If you're the creative type, you could use a cork board, pins, some string and miniature pegs. Pin two strings "wash-line" style across your cork board – one above the other. Move a peg from one line to the other for each milestone or mini-goal you achieve.

- **Gold stars**: It's hard to go past a simple box of gold star stickers. Print out your program, stick it on the fridge and give yourself a gold star for each workout you do or mini-goal you achieve.

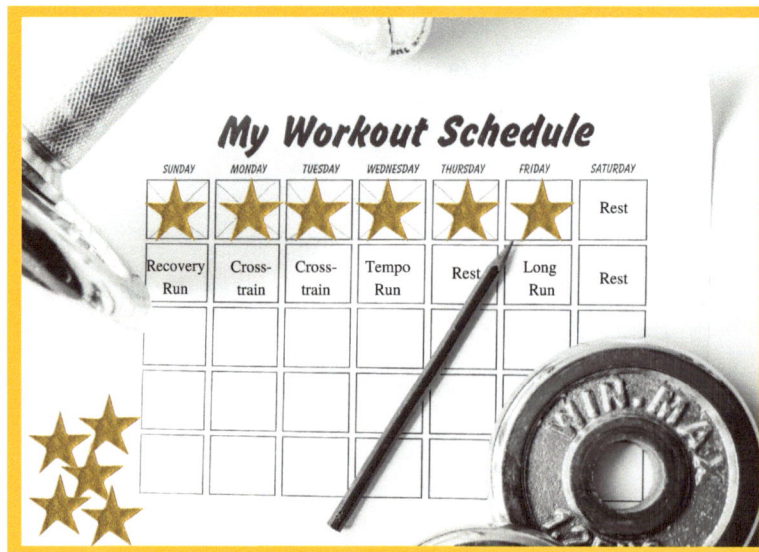

2. Schedule reviews at intervals that align with your milestones

If you have followed our goal-setting tips, your milestones will be specific, measurable, achievable, realistic, and time-based with clear deadlines in place for each milestone. Use these deadlines to schedule short-, mid- and long-term reviews. We recommend weekly, monthly, quarterly (or six monthly), and annual reviews, but you can choose intervals that suit your specific goals.

3. Complete any assessments related to your goals

For example, if you've been following our health and fitness program, use your monthly reviews to completing the wellness and fitness assessments from the Believe section of this book and/or check in with your life coach, nutritionist or fitness professional.

4. Compare your past and current metrics

Your reviews should start with a comparison of your current metrics against your previous and baseline metrics to evaluate your progress. Just bear in mind that this comparison won't give you the full picture...

5. Examine any challenges you faced and how you handled them

To fully understand your metrics, you need to factor in the observations you made regarding any obstacles, stumbling blocks and challenges you've faced, as well as the wins you've had over the review period.

Have you been facing internal challenges such as low energy levels, low mood or lack of motivation? How did they affect your metrics? What can you do to overcome these in future? Revisit the section on reframing and overcoming challenges (pp 62–65) for help.

6. Use your review time to examine your habits

Once a month, once a quarter (or every six months) do a full review of your habits. Have you been able to develop the new habits required to meet your milestones? Are old habits getting in your way? Are there any strategies, such as hypnotherapy, NLP or habit stacking, you could use to break the habits that are sabotaging your progress and replace them with new ones?

Looking at health and fitness goals for example, your monthly review is a great time to read your fitness journal and see how your training and nutrition habits have improved over a four-week period. How many times have you been training each week? Have you been sticking to your nutrtion program? What excuses keep cropping up?

Compare the contents of your fridge and pantry at the start of your program and at monthly intervals along the way. Are you purchasing and eating more natural nutrient-dense foods and fewer sugary, trans-fat-containing foods?

Don't forget the other aspects of your journey, such as mindfulness, sleep, rest, and hydration. Are you practicing mindfulness in your daily life as well as when you eat and train? Have you been honouring your rest days? Are you getting between seven and eight hours of sleep each night? Have you been drinking enough water, and topping up your electrolytes during long training sessions?

7. Be kind to yourself as you examine your progress

Whatever challenges you've been facing, don't spend time beating yourself up about them. Instead, show yourself the same empathy you would show to a friend who was in your situation. Take a positive problem-solving approach and try to find out what you can do to get back on track.

8. Celebrate your successes

While you're reviewing your progress, don't forget to pause and give yourself a pat on the back for each of your successes, no matter how small. Remember you're after progress, not perfection. Every tiny positive change is worth celebrating because it is getting you closer to achieving your goal. We're going to explain exactly how to celebrate and reward yourself for your success in the next chapter, so stay tuned.

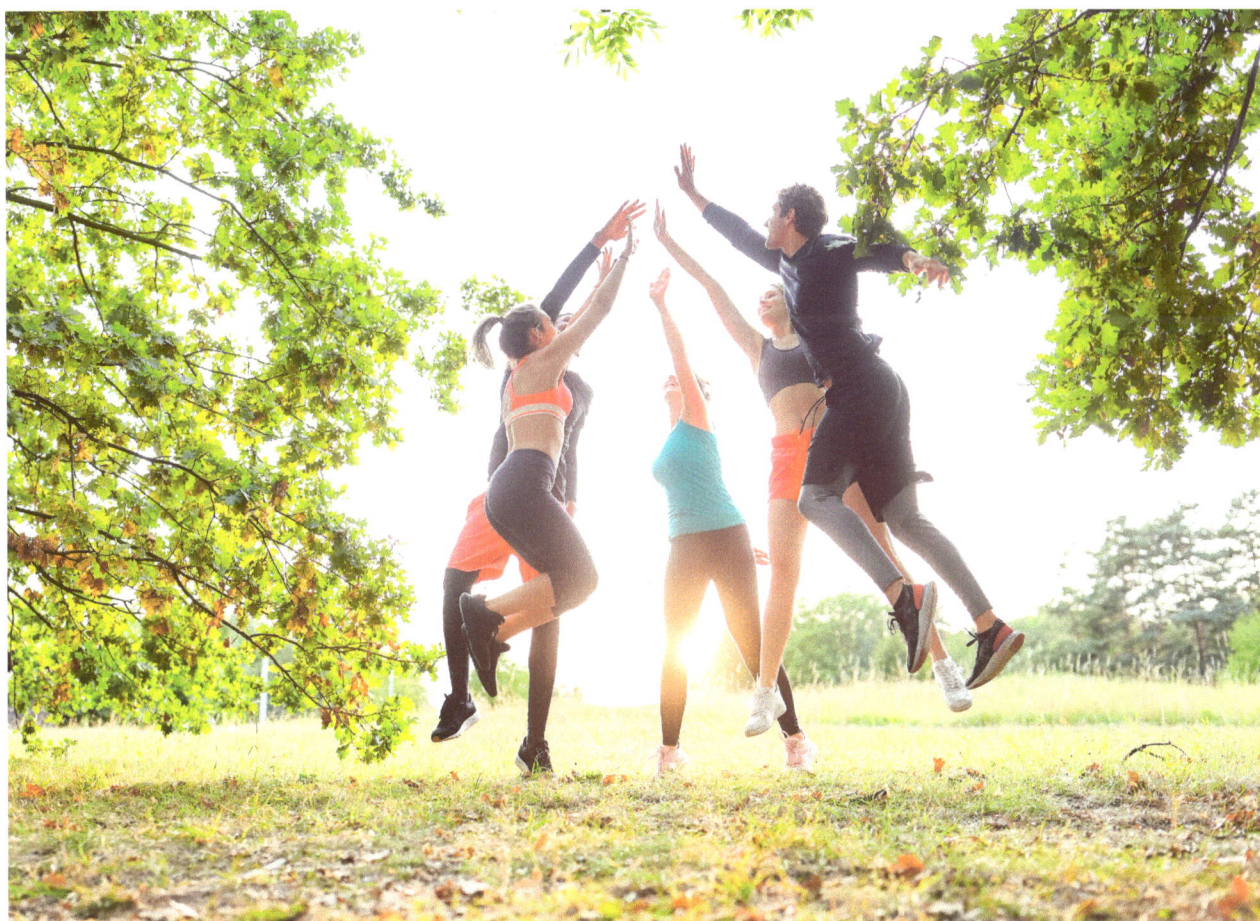

> **66** It's fine to celebrate success, but it is more important to heed the lessons of failure.
>
> Bill Gates

9. Learn from your failures and make positive changes

Progress reviews are not about deciding whether or not you've made the grade. They're about working out how you're going to proceed. Reviewing gives you the opportunity to see how the process of working towards your goals is unfolding in reality – as opposed to how it looked on paper when you first formulated them. It allows you to discover what worked and what didn't. Which goals were easy and which were a struggle. With these new insights, you can make positive changes to your milestones, your overarching plan, and the day-to-day strategies needed to achieve success.

For example, if, after review, you discover that you've been struggling to get to the gym because you've got too much on your plate at the moment, you can use this information to make the changes needed to ensure you still smash your exercise goals. This might mean saying no to some things (e.g., TV, video games or trivia nights) until you reach your fitness goals. It could mean delegating some responsibilities to others at home or at the office. Or, it may simply be a matter of changing the times you go to the gym. Instead of aiming for the 6:30 pm step class, try getting up earlier and going to the 5 am class instead. Can't make any of the classes? Ask the club trainers to provide a weight or cardio program that you can do at a time that suits you. Alternatively, do your workouts at home to save time.

10. Revise your goals

Reviewing your progress also gives you the chance to assess and revise your milestones and your overarching goals. Are these goals still relevant or important to you? Are there other goals you would/should rather be chasing? Perhaps you were a little too ambitious when you initially set your goals, and you need to stretch the timeline out a little? Or circumstances beyond your control have derailed you, and you need to make a fresh start on your journey. Whatever the case, your progress review is the perfect opportunity to decide what's working and what isn't, what to keep and what to change.

11. Revisit the goal setting questions and set new goals

Your quarterly (six monthly) or annual progress reviews are ideal times to set fresh goals.

Use the information in our Goal Setting chapter (pp 51–76) and goal setting questions below to guide you through the process:

- What steps are you going to take to make your goal a reality?
- How much time will you need each day to make this happen?
- What resources or supplies will you need to invest in?
- How much are you willing/able to spend on making this dream a reality?
- What research do you need to do before you get started?
- Can you get help from a group, friend, life coach, nutritionist and/or personal trainer?

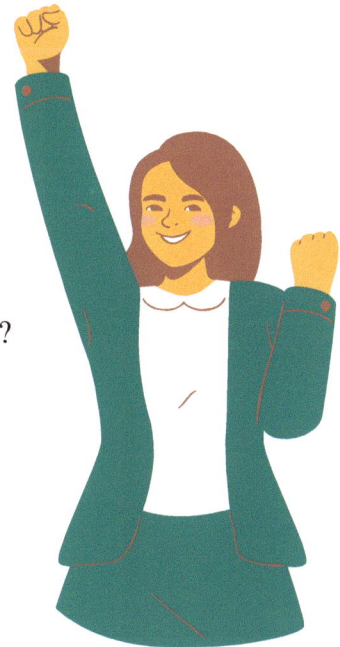

NOTES

Believe. Train. Nourish. Achieve.

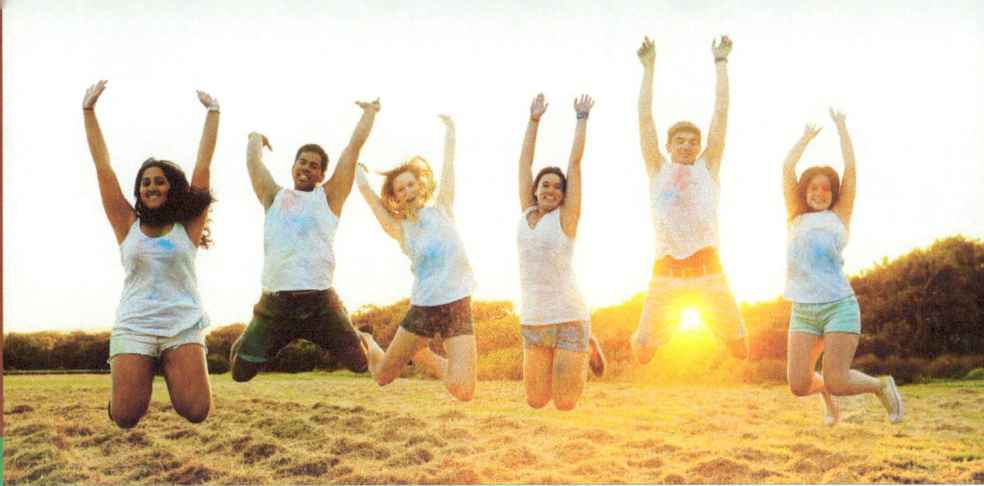

Reward your successes

The more you praise and celebrate your life, the more there is in life to celebrate.

Oprah Winfrey

It is normal, and very human, to criticise and even punish ourselves for "bad behaviour" or to feel guilty for not performing as expected. Whether it's wolfing down that second piece of cake or turning off the alarm and skipping a workout, we're all too eager to beat ourselves up about our failures. But what about those days or weeks when we manage to get up and smash our workouts? When we're strong enough to say no to cakes and lollies? Or when we eat healthy foods and stay hydrated? How often do we take the time to stop and celebrate our successes? Oddly, we're reluctant to give ourselves a pat on the back for accomplishing small victories. We hold back, waiting for that one big achievement, and deny ourselves the benefits that come from celebrating the small successes and milestones along the road to reaching our long-term goals.

Studies indicate that celebrating small wins has a big impact on your overall motivation and success. The sense of accomplishment, no matter how small, boosts your self-esteem, which in turn, helps you to face future tasks with a greater sense of confidence in your own abilities.

The science behind celebrating

Neurologically, celebrating small successes opens up the reward pathway in your brain. In doing so, it activates the release of dopamine, a neurotransmitter that energises your body and lifts your mood, giving you a sense of achievement and pleasure. This triggers a desire to repeat the action that caused the release in the first place. In this way, celebrating your successes (even the small ones) helps you to keep going and motivates you to do even better in future.

How to leverage the power of celebrating your successes

1. Plan your rewards

As you decide on your goals and the daily things that you're going to do to achieve them, make a list of rewards (preferably non-food related) that you can use to celebrate your wins along the way. It's a good idea to include the milestones that will unlock each reward. The bigger the success; the bigger the reward. For example, give yourself a sticker or a gold star every time you complete a daily task, then once you've earned five gold stars, give yourself a reward from your list.

Everyone is unique and will have different ideas about what constitutes a reward. Also, rewards don't always have to cost money, sometimes just taking time off to do something you enjoy can be a reward in itself. Check out our Rewards List for ideas.

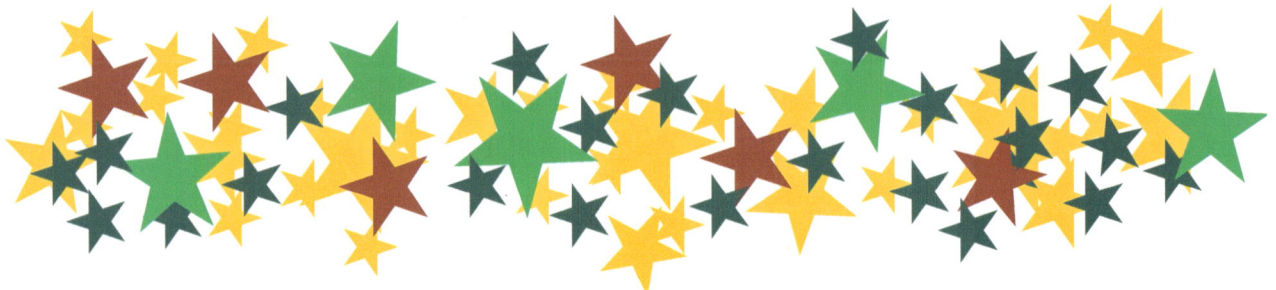

Rewards List

- Spend time on your favourite hobby
- Attend free events in your town
- Spend time with your kids
- Have a family games night
- Take a nap
- Attend a workshop
- Listen to some music
- Plant a garden
- Take a day off work to do as you please
- Read a book from your TBR pile.
- Have a picnic
- Visit an art gallery
- Spend a day lounging beside the pool
- Go to the beach
- Go for a walk in nature
- Share your progress on social media and soak up the kudos
- Arrange a coffee date and tell a friend about your achievements
- Grab your phone or camera and take some photos of cityscapes
- Wander through the botanical gardens
- Enjoy a massage/float session
- Get a mani/pedicure
- Go to the hairdresser
- Get a facial
- Go see a movie
- Stream a movie you've always wanted to watch
- Go op-shopping or window-shopping
- Buy a new fitness outfit
- Buy a new dress/suit
- Treat yourself to art classes
- Try your hand at a craft e.g., candle-making, mosaics or resin-art
- Buy a new handbag or shoes
- Buy something nice for your home
- Buy a new watch or fitness tracker
- Buy new running shoes or trainers
- Book a personal training session
- Go to a yoga/pilates class
- Learn to play an instrument
- Give yourself a home spa day
- Ride your bicycle
- Make a new workout playlist

2. Act like an ant

Did you know that a colony of ants can move 50 tons of dirt in a single year – one tiny grain at a time? That's because ants understand the accumulative power that comes from tiny acts repeated consistently.

Acting like an ant means breaking your goals down into daily tasks and doing these little daily tasks consistently to achieve big things. And, most importantly, you'll be celebrating the successful achievement of each of these daily tasks, no matter how small, because they will lead you to achieve great things.

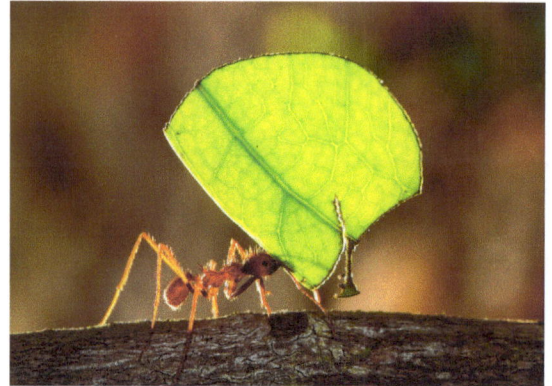

3. Track your progress

We've mentioned the importance of tracking your progress and explained ways to do it, what we may not have mentioned is that you can use your tracking devices to set reminders that will prompt you to stop and celebrate your progress. Nifty, right?

4. Set aside time to reflect on your progress and reward your successes

It's easy to get so caught up in chasing your goals that you forget to take time out to celebrate your successes. The best way to ensure that you get the reward you planned when achieving your milestones, and benefit from the energy and renewed motivation that comes with celebrating your successes, is to deliberately set time aside to review your progress and celebrate your victories. Be sure to schedule weekly, monthly, quarterly/six monthly and annual *review and reward* days.

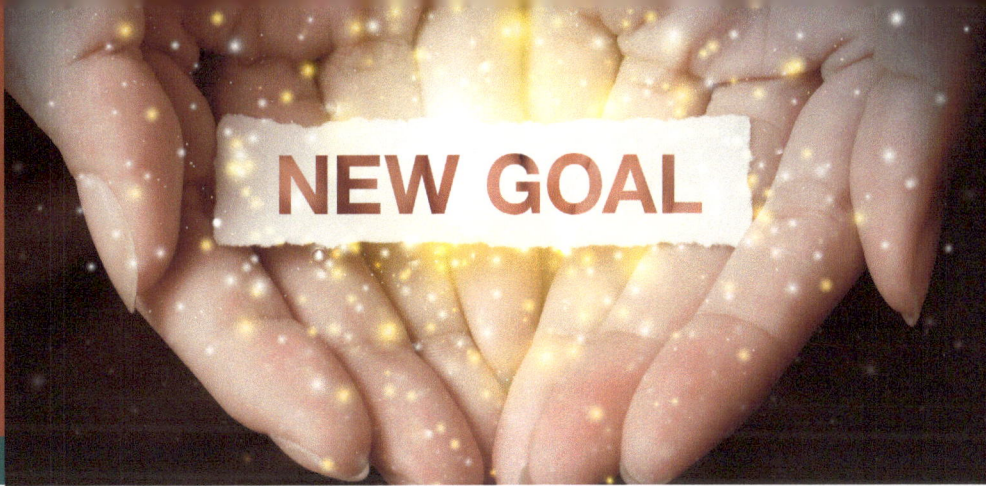

NEW GOAL

Renew your goals

Renew your intentions, reaffirm your goals, and strive tirelessly

and be steadfast in achieving them.

Islamic Proverb

The old saying "life is about the journey and not the destination" may be a cliché, but it's true nonetheless. And, if you look at life from this perspective, it's easy to see how important it is to keep moving forward, setting new goals, and achieving them.

The process of becoming the best version of yourself is extremely rewarding and exciting, but it is hardly ever straightforward. It is challenging. It takes courage, determination, time, and commitment.

There may be times when the going gets tough, but there will also be times of great joy and a sense of accomplishment when you achieve the success you've worked for.

It's vital to take time out along the way to review and renew your intentions, reaffirm your commitment, and set new goals for yourself.

Reset and renew your goals regularly

Aim to do smaller reviews weekly or once a month, bigger ones every quarter or every six months, and a major review once a year. Include all your goals (health, financial, professional/career, personal, relationship) in your reviews. Take a moment to consider how you're tracking. What (if anything) has stood in the way of achieving your goals? What has helped you to achieve them? Then decide on the next steps by asking these simple questions.

1. Do you want to take any of your goals a step further?

For example, if your goal was to lose 5 kg in six months, and you've achieved that. Do you want to reset that goal and lose another 5 kg in the next six months?

2. Are there goals where you just need a "do-over"?

If your goal was to pay off your debts, but the circumstances beyond your control made this impossible, can you renew that goal and start working towards it afresh in the coming months?

3. Are all these goals still relevant or important to you?

Especially if you're feeling overwhelmed by all your goals, this might be a good time to trim them down to a more manageable list. Identify the ones that no longer resonate and let them go. If you're up to replacing them with others, ask what other goals you would/should rather be chasing. For example, if your goal was to learn to play the ukulele, but you never take the time to practice, and you're finding it less enjoyable than you first thought it would be. Maybe it's time to put the ukulele aside and sign up for that French cooking class you've been dreaming about instead?

4. Are some of your goals a little overambitious?

If you're struggling to live up to the demands of some of your bigger goals, you could try breaking them down into smaller, more achievable goals that will keep you motivated.

For example, if you made it a goal to follow a strictly vegan diet this year, but you have not been able to stick to it, you could break that goal down into a more manageable one by making it your goal to follow a strictly vegan diet one or two days per week. Once you've managed to make this small change, you will build momentum, which makes it easier to increase your goal to eating vegan three days per week and so on.

Recharge

Use your goal reviewing times to remind yourself to take time out from chasing your goals to simply relax and reenergise your mind and body.

Treat yourself to a massage, enjoy a stroll around some local parks, take the family out for a picnic or lie in your hammock and read a good book.

Whatever represents rest and relaxation to you – do it regularly.

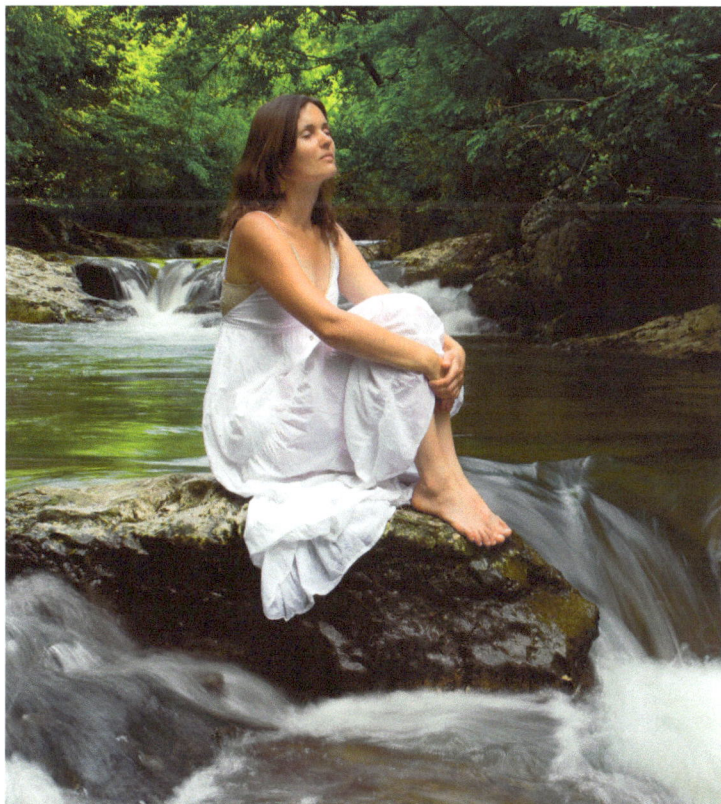

NOTES

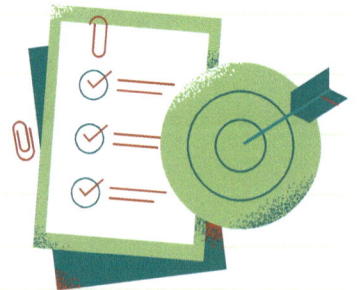

Believe. Train. Nourish. Achieve.

CONCLUSION

Thank you for coming along on this journey with us. We hope you enjoyed learning about ways to start living your best, healthiest, and most fulfilling life.

We sincerely hope that this book offers more than just a great read. We hope that it becomes a well-worn and much-loved companion that will guide your progress towards the sense of peace and fulfillment that comes with the alignment of mind and body.

Whatever you do, please don't forget our motto: progress, not perfection. Be patient with yourself as you learn and grow. Take things slowly, and don't beat yourself up if you fail. Learn from your failures and move on.

Before signing off, we'd like to thank you again for purchasing this book, and, in doing so, supporting Rosie's Friends on the Street (https://rosies.org.au/).

If you have enjoyed reading the book, please tell your friends about it and leave a review on the bookseller's website.

If you would like help and/or advice on mindset, goal setting, healthy eating, fitness, and techniques such as neurolinguistic programming, clinical hypnosis, and life coaching to help you create a life you love, please get in touch.

Jo, Johnny & Mandy

www.platinummindandbody.com

Acknowledgments

The authors would like to thank Fred van Staden, Marie Palframan, and Jane McCarthy for proofreading the manuscript.

A special word of thanks goes to Michael Chandler for his patience and support throughout the writing, designing, editing, and publishing of this book. Thanks for believing in possibilities.

Author's note: As far as possible, I have tried to attribute every quote in this book to it's original source. There were however a few that eluded me, no matter how much I searched. If one of these is yours, I apologise. Please contact me, and I will update text.

www.ingramcontent.com/pod-product-compliance
Lightning Source LLC
Chambersburg PA
CBHW061134030426
42334CB00003B/34